the Worrywart's Companion

Twenty-One Ways to Soothe
Yourself and Worry Smart

Other Books by Docpotter

the Worrywart's Companion

Twenty-One Ways to Soothe Yourself and Worry Smart

BEVERLY POTTER, PH.D.

New York Chicago San Francisco Lisbon London Madrid Mexico City
Milan New Delhi San Juan Seoul Singapore Sydney Toronto

The **McGraw·Hill** *Companies*

Library of Congress Cataloging-in-Publication Data

Potter, Beverly A.
    The worrywart's companion : twenty-one ways to soothe yourself and worry
smart / by Beverly Potter.
        p.   cm.
    Includes bibliographical references and index.
    ISBN 978-0-07-160213-6 (alk. paper)
    1. Worry.   2. Anxiety.   I. Title.

BF575.W8P684   2009
152.4'6—dc22   2008008734

1 2 3 4 5 6 7 8 9 10 11 12 13 14 15 16 17 18 19 20   DOC/DOC   0 9 8

ISBN   978-0-07-160213-6
MHID   0-07-160213-5

Interior illustration copyright © Susan Gross
Interior design by Susan H. Hartman

McGraw-Hill books are available at special quantity discounts to use as premiums
and sales promotions or for use in corporate training programs. To contact a
representative, please visit the Contact Us pages at www.mhprofessional.com.

This book is printed on acid-free paper.

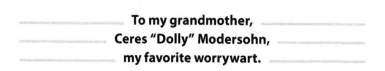

**To my grandmother,
Ceres "Dolly" Modersohn,
my favorite worrywart.**

CONTENTS

PART 1   What Is Worrywarting?

PART 2   How to Worry Smarter

PART 3   Twenty-One Ways to Soothe Yourself and Worry Smart

If you feel distressed or unable to cope with worrisome events, you should consult with a qualified counselor, therapist, or clergy. The ideas, procedures, and suggestions contained in this book are intended to inform, teach, and encourage but should not be substituted for consulting with a physician or therapist. If you are utilizing counseling services, please ask your counselor or therapist to review this book and follow his or her advice in implementing any self-change procedures.

ACKNOWLEDGMENTS

Awarm thank-you to all the people who helped me better understand worry. Special thanks to Julie Bennett, who conceived of this book and pressed me to write it. I want to express my appreciation to Pamela Butler for her work on "the language of self-support"; to Lucinda Bassett for her wonderfully informative tapes on panic and what to do about it; to Edward de Bono for his clear thoughts on thinking; to C. W. Metcalf for his many ways of getting benefit from humor; and to Peter Goleman, whose fascinating work on emotional intelligence inspired the concept of "smart worry."

I owe a great deal of thanks to Sebastian, who never stopped encouraging me and, like a good trouper, spent hours assembling delightful quotes to inspire and entertain you.

Last, but never least, I thank you, my readers, for taking this little book home with you. If you find comfort in it when you feel a worry coming on, then all my work will have been worth it. Thanks, friends!

What Is Heaven? What Is Hell?

After traveling for thirty days, a Seeker finally arrived at the Shaman Woman's mountain cabin. She was sitting on a small stool in front and looked up as the Seeker spoke. "Shaman Woman, I have traveled from a distant land to ask you an important question."

"What is it you seek?" the Shaman asked.

"Would you explain the concepts of heaven and hell?" the Seeker inquired.

"You are a foolish child. I have no time for such silly questions. Come back when you have a question of substance to ask!" the Shaman retorted in contempt, as she waved the Seeker away.

Distraught, the Seeker began pacing back and forth. "What did I say wrong?" the Seeker worried aloud. "I've offended the Shaman Woman. How could I have acted so poorly? What can I do? I can't go home without an answer. What will people in my village think? I'll never be able to face them again."

"That," said the Shaman Woman, "is hell."

Surprised at hearing the Shaman speak, the Seeker stopped pacing. Realizing the truth in the wise woman's words, the Seeker calmed down, bowed, and thanked her. "Yes, Wise One," the Seeker said. "I see now that my mind running on wildly makes life hell. I feel quite better now that I stopped nagging myself."

"And that," said the Shaman Woman, "is heaven."

PART 1

What Is Worrywarting?

CHAPTER 1

Worrywarting Is Hell

The mind is its own place, and in itself can make a heaven of hell, a hell of heaven.

—JOHN MILTON

The job of worry is to anticipate danger before it arises and identify possible perils, to come up with ways to lessen the risks, and to rehearse what you plan to do. Worrywarts get stuck in identifying danger as they immerse themselves in the dread associated with the threat, which may be real or, more likely, imagined. They spin out an endless loop of melodrama, blowing everything out of proportion. "What if I have a heart attack?" "What if there is an earthquake?" "What if someone breaks in when I'm asleep?"

While worrywarts insist worrying is helpful, little is solved. Stuck in thinking ruts, they stop living in the here and now—the present moment. Worrywarting is torment—a kind of self-imposed purgatory that makes you feel bad, stresses you out, and wastes precious moments of your life.

Worse yet, worry begets more worry, setting into motion a vicious circle of frightening thoughts and anxious response. It is self-perpetuating, pushing into greater anxiety and more worry. Allowed to continue unchecked, chronic worry can evolve into panic attacks and, in extreme cases, agoraphobia, which is a paralyzing fear of having a panic attack, especially in public. It can be so severe that, in the worst cases, the sufferer can't leave home.

Are You a Worrywart?

You probably wonder sometimes whether you are the only person in the world plagued with worrying. Do you think of yourself as a worrywart? A lot of people do. Taking the quiz presented here will help you better understand what worry-warting is and whether or not you are one.

Worrywart Quiz

Instructions: Thinking of how you usually feel and usually handle situations, rate how much each statement is like you. Use a scale from 1 to 9, with 1 representing "not at all like me" and 9 representing "very much like me." After you've rated each statement, add up your score to see if you are a worrywart.

SCALE

| NOT AT ALL LIKE ME | 1 | 2 | 3 | 4 | 5 | 6 | 7 | 8 | 9 | VERY MUCH LIKE ME |

Physical Anxiety

_____ **1.** Worrying makes me restless and jumpy.

_____ **2.** I get tense and uptight when worrying.

_____ **3.** My heart races when I worry.

_____ **4.** Worrying causes a tightness in my chest.

Emotional Reactivity

_____ **5.** I react strongly to things.

_____ **6.** I react first and think second.

_____ **7.** Anxiety seems to come from nowhere.

_____ **8.** I often overreact.

Social Anxiety

_____ **9.** I worry about what I "should" do.

_____ **10.** I worry about what others think.

_____ **11.** I feel guilty about things.

_____ **12.** I worry about being alone.

Catastrophic Thinking

_____ **13.** I imagine the worst that could happen.

_____ **14.** Many of my worries begin with "What if . . . ?"

_____ **15.** I worry that something terrible will happen.

_____ **16.** I notice negatives in most situations.

Obsessive Thinking

_____ **17.** My thoughts race from one worry to another.

_____ **18.** Sometimes the kind of thing I worry about scares me.

_____ **19.** When I worry I have a one-track mind.

_____ **20.** I'm afraid to not worry.

Judgmental Thinking

_____ **21.** I worry when things are not done the way they "should" be done.

_____ **22.** I'm a perfectionist.

_____ **23.** I worry about small flaws and errors.

_____ **24.** I worry about doing well enough.

Controlling

_____ **25.** I worry about being calm and in control.

_____ **26.** I worry about going crazy.

_____ **27.** People think of me as a "strong" person.

_____ **28.** I'm unable to control my worrying.

Hypervigilance

_____ **29.** I am on guard.

_____ **30.** I pay attention to anything irregular.

_____ **31.** I'm very watchful, even when resting or playing.

_____ **32.** I like things to be predictable.

Dysfunctional Behavior

_____ **33.** Worries keep me awake at night.

_____ **34.** Worrying interferes with my life.

_____ **35.** I avoid things that I worry about.

_____ **36.** I worry myself sick.

SCORING

36–126   *Not a worrywart:* You do not become entrapped in senseless worry. You have a head start in becoming a smart worrier because you don't have to overcome obsessive worrying.

127–234 *Worrywart potential:* You have a moderate tendency to worry, which, unchecked, could progress to worrywarting. However, you have an excellent chance of becoming a smarter worrier if you begin now.

235–324 *You are a worrywart:* You are hooked on worry—almost like a drug. Worrying is detracting from the quality of your life. But you can become a smart worrier with determination and hard work. With each step life will become fuller.

Make a note of your score in a personal notebook or journal and keep it for future reference. (As you read on you'll learn how to use a personal journal as a powerful tool for transforming worrywarting into smart worry.) Pay particular attention to items you rated 7, 8, and 9. After trying out some of the techniques in this book, you might find it interesting to take the quiz again and compare the scores.

Worrywarting Is Reinforcing

Worrying is reinforcing in the same way as superstition. Like an amulet carried to ward off some anticipated danger, worry is credited with preventing bad things from happening. It is like the story of two women, one of whom is waving her arms about. When a second woman asks what she is doing, the first woman replies, "I'm keeping the tigers away." When the second woman observes, "But there aren't any tigers around here," the first woman answers triumphantly, "You see, it's working!"

Like superstitious behavior, worry gives momentary relief and actually reduces anxiety. At first, when you worry and disaster doesn't happen, you experience a sense of relief that credits the worry with preventing the disaster. In the previous example, when the tigers didn't come, the woman experienced relief that she associated with waving her arms. Once the pattern is learned, the act of waving arms relieves anxiety. The same dynamic is at work with worry. Once the worrywart habit is learned, worrying provides the worrier a sense of relief from anxiety. Research on chronic worriers shows that when worriers are immersed in worry they don't notice physical sensations of the anxiety triggered by the worry and so experience a sense of relief. Of course, as we know, the relief is short-lived. Worrying masks anxiety temporarily but doesn't do anything to correct the worrisome situation. Chronic worry stirs up ever more things to fear, renewing the very anxiety that it was to dispel.

You Can Break Free of Worrywarting

If you are a worrywart, don't despair. There is hope. There is something you can do, beginning today, to change from being a worrywart to *learning* to worry smart. The important word here is learning. You are not a born worrier. You learned to worry. You will not be admonished to "stop worrying." Worrying is helpful—when it is done effectively. You will discover what it means to worry smart and how to become a smart worrier.

CHAPTER 2

Worrywarts Go to Extremes

In the night, imagining some fear,
How easy is a bush supposed a bear.
—WILLIAM SHAKESPEARE, *A Midsummer Night's Dream*

Worriers come in all ages, from all walks of life, and in both sexes. We all worry sometimes. But worrywarts worry a lot—frequently to the point where it gets in the way of living. People who have high anxiety levels tend to be worrywarts. While we usually think of women as being more prone to worrying, men can be world-class worriers. Women tend to talk their worries over with friends, while men are more likely to keep their worries to themselves. Children, too, starting as early as five or six years old, can be worriers.

Worrywarts "Catastrophize"

Worrywarts catastrophize—"Oh no! What if?"—and conjure up one frightening situation after another, most of which have almost no chance of happening. Instead of developing a plan for averting the threatening event, like deer who freeze in the lights of an oncoming car, worrywarts become paralyzed by their own scary thoughts bearing down on them. Their minds fix on a frightening improbable possibility, replaying it again and again in their imagination, until it becomes a very believable pending catastrophe.

Jody often lies awake at night imaging awful "what if" scenarios. "Sometimes I worry what if I get really sick and I die. I lay awake imagining my funeral. I picture my husband standing by my casket and think about his finding another woman. Then I wonder who she would be and if he already knows her, as I go through all the women I know one by one, picturing each with Jim. I'm so tired in the morning that Jim has to drive the kids to school, making him late for work, so he's furious at me. So I worry about that all day."

Is There a Worm in Your Tea?

The Seeker and Shaman Woman were sitting under a grape arbor having tea on a bright sunny afternoon. "It's a lovely afternoon," remarked the Shaman, as she soaked in the sun's warmth.

Frowning, the Seeker said, "Yeah, I guess so," apparently oblivious to the magic of the perfect day.

"You are worrying again," observed the Shaman.

"What makes me worry so much, Shaman Woman?" asked the Seeker.

"It's like a worm in your tea," answered the Shaman.

Only half listening, "Yeah, I guess," the Seeker replied politely, lost in his thoughts.

"Would you like some warm tea?" asked the Shaman as she poured a cup and handed it to the Seeker.

Thanking the Shaman, the Seeker absently took the cup. Just as he was about to take a sip, he looked into the cup and to his horror saw a worm in his tea. "Ugh, there's a worm in my tea. This is terrible! How awful! What if I didn't see the worm and drank the tea? What could have happened? I might have been poisoned. I could have died!" The Seeker went on and on, becoming increasingly upset as he did.

"Is that a worm in your tea," asked the Shaman as she pointed to a grapevine above the Seeker's head, "or is it a reflection that you see?"

Worrywarts Are Constantly Vigilant

Worrywarts are constantly vigilant. With uneasy apprehension they watch for small signs of danger, which they magnify into pending doom, overestimating the odds of their occurrence. Jody is an example. "If there is one thing I worry about most it is getting sick. When I notice a sensation in my body I concentrate on it, analyzing each twinge. It is not unusual for me to lie awake all night, terrified and convinced that the pounding of my heart is signaling a heart attack."

Worrywarts Analyze Everything

Worrywarts analyze everything to ferret out negative possibilities. Like a dog working over a bone, the worrywart bites and rips at the worrisome notion. When a risk is uncovered, he or she tears into it, ripping away to get to the central danger.

Jody's husband, Jim, for example, worries about his income-tax return, which he prepared himself for the first time. "I get to worrying about the return I prepared and calculating the odds of being audited. I review each deduction I took and rehearse my defenses to the auditor. In the process, I think of another potential vulnerability and start all over again."

Worrywarts Are Perfectionists

Worrywarts expect perfection, especially with respect to their own performance. They push themselves to achieve at very high levels, criticize small flaws, and overlook progress. Not too surprisingly, worrywarts spend a lot of time worrying about starting, performing, and the possibility of failing at it.

Because of their high standards, worrywarts are usually competent, dependable doers. The problem is that having higher expectations of themselves than they would have of other people, they drive themselves relentlessly, all the while worrying that they won't make the grade. Thinking is no longer balanced so that irrational ideas are accepted unquestioningly. Events are right or wrong, fair or unfair, black or white.

Worrywarts Are Emotionally Sensitive

Worrywarts are especially sensitive to other people's needs, often becoming overly concerned about keeping other people happy, sometimes to their own detriment. They tend to take things personally, often overreacting as they worry about being rejected even when there is no evidence of disapproval.

Worry Is Not Good or Bad

Worry, itself, is not good or bad. Everyone worries. Not only is worrying normal, but it is a survival skill—if you worry smart. Like many things, it is a matter of degree. Too little worry is not good because you don't pay attention, so you miss seeing problems coming when you still have time to take action. Too much worry—worrywarting—is not good either because you get stuck in exaggerated fears that overload your system, as life passes you by.

Like worrywarts, smart worriers look for dangers and analyze risks. But unlike worrywarts, smart worriers move on to problem solving when a risk is identified. When there is nothing that can be done at the moment, which is so often the case, smart worriers use a variety of techniques to keep their minds off the worrisome situation and soothe themselves until taking action is possible.

CHAPTER 3

Worrywarting Is a Style of Thinking

Life is 10 percent what you make it and 90 percent how you take it.

—ANONYMOUS

You continually create your personal view of the world with what you think. Thoughts interpret information from the senses, set your expectations, and frame your vision. Worrywarting is a mental habit, a pattern of thinking that limits self-confidence. By parading threatening possibilities before you, it makes you want to pull back. Habits *can* be changed. It is hard to do, but with an understanding of how thoughts work, a few techniques, and the motivation to become a smart worrier, changing thinking habits is a liberating challenge.

Automatic Self-Talk

Most of us experience thinking as a sort of silent talk or monologue we tell ourselves, what psychologists call "self-talk." Usually you don't notice your self-talk because it goes on automatically in a process called automatic thinking. Automatic thoughts are a kind of shorthand, with one or two words conveying the entire meaning about a situation. They are irrational fleeting thoughts like "always losing" or "gotta hurry" or "no love for me." What worrywarts tell themselves can be contrary to factual evidence, as well as being overgeneralized, absolutist, one-sided, and dogmatic.

Yet, self-talk *sounds like* the truth—to you inside your mind, talking to yourself. So thoughts driven by expectations and prejudices go unchallenged. Worrywarts accept things they say to themselves that they would never accept if someone else said them.

How Your Brain Is Wired

CT scans of working brains have shown that thoughts record a "neurosignature." The more you think a particular thought the more indelible becomes the signature, sort of like a fingerprint. Learned pathways are created by repetitive thoughts, which cause impulses to continually retrace certain neural paths until following that circuit becomes virtually automatic, locking you into habitual patterns of thinking and behaving. It's a form of self-conditioning that goes on without awareness. This "soft-wiring" is a circular thing where emotions and personality actually influence biology—literally building neural pathways in the brain—and, in turn, biology influences emotion, creating a tremendous potential for negative cycles to set into motion. And this is just what happens with worrywarts. Something starts you worrying, which in turn triggers anxiety, leading to more worrisome thoughts. As you worry, the habitual neural pathway is reinforced, making it easier to move along it in the future, instead of forging a new one. If you do this enough with a particular train of thought, it becomes automatic. No wonder you can get stuck.

How You Talk to Yourself Is Learned

As you grow up, self-talk is learned from interacting with significant adults—your parents, teachers, older siblings. Dr. Pamela Butler, author of *Talking to Yourself: Learning the Language of Self-Support*, says if the influential people in your early life were harsh, critical, or judgmental, or if they were fearful and constantly warned you of dangers, you have probably incorporated these characteristics into your self-talk.

If you are a worrywart, and you probably are if you are reading this book, your self-talk is filled with judgments and criticism. You would probably never talk to a friend with the same harshness that you use when talking to yourself. If you were talking to a friend, you would probably be reassuring and challenge the severity of your friend's self-criticisms, yet you hammer away at yourself.

You Feel the Way You Think

Fortunately, your brain has a tremendous capacity for adapting—what psychologists call "plasticity." This means that your soft-wiring is malleable because it is learned. Change the way you think, and your picture of the world changes, the way you act and feel changes—your life changes. Sound like a dramatic claim? The fact is: *you feel the way you think!* Negative feelings like anxiety, depression, and anger don't actually result from the bad things that happen; they result from the way you think about those events.

Except for responses to physical pain like pulling back quickly when touching a hot stove, an event in and of itself doesn't cause you to respond. Events are just events. If you observe yourself in slow motion, when something upsetting happens, you will notice that it is the judgment you make about the event that triggers your response. Suppose, for example, someone cuts you off while driving on the freeway, and you think to yourself, "Boy, what a jerk! The nerve of that guy. He could have caused an accident. What he did was really wrong. I could have been driven off the road and gotten hurt!" By this time you feel angry and indignant. But it wasn't the driver cutting you off that triggered your anger. It was what you told yourself about it that made you angry.

Things happen and worrywarts tell themselves, "This is awful. This shouldn't happen to me. This is a disaster." Then they respond to those catastrophic thoughts, not to the event. It is not the event itself that directly causes or creates your feelings. It's the judgments that trigger disappointment, fear, anxiety, anger, and other emotions. You constantly judge life—draw conclusions—then respond to these judgments as if they were objective reality. It's hard to find something that the mind regards with complete impartiality because there is always a judgment, however mild, a liking or a disliking. Judgments happen in a fraction of a second, without your realizing it, and you respond to these judgmental thoughts, not to the event. This occurs so quickly that you're rarely aware that you lead your life by what you say to yourself about things that happen and not what actually happens to you.

Distorted Thinking

Psychologists have found that when people are extremely anxious, fearful, angry, or feeling other emotional disturbance, their self-talk is usually irrational, exaggerated, selective, and unrealistic, filled with shoulds, oughts, musts, what-ifs, generalizations, all-or-nothing thinking, and blame. This type of thinking is oppressive. The famous psychotherapist Karen Horney said that most people tend to rule themselves by the "tyranny of the shoulds." You build ideal pictures of the future with shoulds—the way the world should be, the way others should be, and the way you should be. When things don't conform to your notion of the way it should be, your idealized castles in the sky come tumbling down. You tell yourself that it is awful and the emotional brain interprets it as a crisis—a threat—and sounds the alarm. Extreme anxiety, even panic, can result, and it gets attributed to the event rather than the shoulds you were telling yourself.

Thinking Habits

We tend to think that thoughts are some sort of ethereal process that goes on outside our control. But actually, thoughts are behaviors—internal behaviors—that go on inside, that only you can observe. Thinking is something you do—it's a habit. Habits are automatic behaviors. Worrywarts have some bad thinking habits. You were not born with a predisposition to anxious self-talk. You learned it! You can change bad thinking habits in the same way you would change any other habit.

You can master your thoughts rather than go on being enslaved by them. Worrywarting is the mind run amok—out of control like a wild elephant. You don't have to stop worrying to break free. You can take charge of your worrying—when you worry, how you worry, what you worry about, how long you worry, and what you do next. Smart worriers think about the negatives and dangers of a situation, just as worrywarts do, but once they have worried the problem through, they change how they think about it; they let the worry go and redirect their thinking to finding a solution.

We'll look more closely at ways to worry smarter in Part 2. Before we do that, let's consider some other aspects of worrywarting, because understanding how we worry now can help to learn to worry in a new and smarter way.

CHAPTER 4

Worrywarts Let Emotions Take Over

Don't lose your head
To gain a minute
You need your head
Your brains are in it.

—Burma-Shave, *1963 roadside ad*

You have two minds, a "rational mind" that ponders and reflects, analyzes and plans; and an "emotional mind," which is intuitive and reactive, not logical. In normal daily discourse, thoughts precede feelings as the rational mind takes the lead, planning, coordinating, thinking, and calling on the emotional mind for intuition and wisdom. In an emergency, however, this balance of power shifts rapidly as the emotional brain takes over.

The Emotional Mind Reacts Fast

Under emergency conditions impulses take a neurological "back door" directly into the emotional brain, which is a faster circuit that allows instant action and can mean the difference between life and death. This survival mechanism enables you to react fast to get out of the way. Thanks to the super capabilities of the emotional brain, all of this occurs in a split second—before you can think about it. Respond first, think second.

The power of the emotional mind saved me from certain terror one night. After visiting friends for a couple of hours, I was returning to the car, which was parked along the street under a pine tree. Just as I leaned down to open the door, I suddenly became aware that there was something an inch or two from my cheek. Instantly, without effort, my body propelled itself several feet back from the car as I yelled, "Oh, my gawd! Oh, my gawd!" But I didn't know what it was that had terrified me until I heard myself screaming, "It's a spider. It's a spider!" Only then did I realize that the most enormous garden spider I'd ever seen, measuring at least four inches from gigantic claw to gigantic claw, was hanging on a web stretched from a tree branch to the door handle of my car. The thought of that spider on my cheek or down my neck makes me appreciate—and marvel at—that wonderful ability to trust my instincts, reacting immediately without hesitation.

What Happens When You Worry

There is, however, a downside to this swift reactivity. When the alarm sounds, the emotional brain takes over, recruiting the rest of the brain to its urgent agenda. Reactions are so fast that it is easy to jump to conclusions and act before you have full confirming evidence. If people say to you, "You overreacted!" "You lost it!" or "You blew it!" they usually are referring to the experience of your emotions gaining the upper hand, swamping the rational mind. Daniel Goleman, in his fascinating book *Emotional Intelligence*, calls these moments of irrational behavior "emotional hijacking." This is what happened to a police officer who shot a teenager one night because he thought the kid had drawn a gun, which turned out to be a paper bag that looked like a gun in the dim light.

Your mind tells your body what is going on, which means that if you think the worrisome situation is a catastrophe, your body believes there is a real emergency. Worry sounds the alarm, and the back door to the emotional brain opens. Hormones are secreted, readying you to fight or to flee the threat. Your attention is riveted on the source of fear, overriding rational thought as your memory systems retrieve information from the emotional brain relevant to the emergency.

To the emotional brain, an emergency is an emergency. It doesn't matter whether there is a real danger standing before you—a robber with a gun saying, "Your money or your life!"—or only a worry about a *possible* danger—"*What if* a robber holds me up?" By the time the neural impulse goes through the back door to your emotional brain, both become emergencies. "Is there a threat?" your vigilant inner eye asks. "Yes! It's an emergency!" your worrying mind answers, triggering the same mechanism that allowed me to avoid a spider on my neck, and that lead to someone shooting a teenager armed only with a paper bag.

When you worrywart, you keep yourself in a chronic state of low-grade emotional hijacking that physically stresses you and diminishes your ability to think clearly. Your performance suffers because worry colors your judgment, so you may act in ways that you normally would not. Worry clouds your logic as you work yourself into taking extreme positions you would reject when cool-headed. Worry interferes with your ability to learn and prejudices how you view situations.

You become reactive, emotions overriding your rational capabilities. Of course you *think*, but your thinking is driven by emotion, not reason. You convince yourself that doom is about to descend upon you at any moment. Rose Anne's worrying about her house is an example of how worrywarting diminishes quality of life: "I was planning some work to be done on the foundation of my 100-year-old home, which is built on a steep hillside, and I was really nervous about it. I had heard stories of foundations being opened to reveal more problems so that the cost doubled. The night before the contractor showed up to begin work, Tom and I went to a movie, but instead of watching the movie, I had a movie of my own in my mind as I envisioned the contractor opening up the walls and discovering that all the joists had been eaten away by termites. I realized about halfway through the movie that I hadn't heard a single word of it."

Rose Anne worked herself up needlessly over something that wasn't very likely, and at a time when she couldn't do anything about it. She deprived herself of the enjoyment of the movie. Instead, she came out of the theater in a near panic. The images of disaster that Rose Anne created and her ability to actually see her catastrophic images are remarkable, but these desirable abilities are being employed destructively.

As a smart worrier, Rose Anne would catch herself dwelling on useless worry, like imagining massive termite damage under her floorboards, and redirect her attention outward to the movie. She would additionally soothe herself by breathing deeply, and, talking to herself like a supportive friend would, she would challenge her wild worries.

CHAPTER 5

Worrywarts Worry Themselves Sick

I highly recommend worrying. It is much more effective than dieting.

—WILLIAM POWELL

L ike a mantra, worrywarts silently chant their fears, but unlike a mantra that brings serenity, worrywarting generates anxiety and revs up the body. The emotional mind reacts to imagined catastrophes as if they were real by sending signals to the body that there is a danger—a threat—and the body mobilizes to ready for it. Noticing tension, the emotional mind triggers more anxiety and worry, setting into motion a cycle of escalating worry and anxiety.

Emotions and Disease

The emotional mind interprets worrisome situations that stir up feelings of being victimized, helpless, and out of control as "threatening." Faced with a threat, the body mobilizes to prepare to fight or to flee. Blood pressure and blood sugar levels go up, digestion slows, breathing becomes shallow, muscles contract, the heart pounds. Nonessential bodily functions shut down; only those essential for survival keep operating. You are ready to take action, to confront a life-threatening event. But you are not facing a life-threatening event—you are worrywarting, creating exaggerated images in your mind of disasters that your emotional brain responds to as if they were real. Medical literature indicates that people who are chronically anxious, who suffer long periods of sadness and pessimism, who experience unremitting tension or incessant hostility, or who are cynical or suspicious have a dramatically greater risk of developing diseases, including asthma, arthritis, headaches, peptic ulcers, and heart disease. Worrywarting, which keeps you in a state of anxiety, also puts you at risk.

Worrying Triggers Negative Emotions

Most people don't realize the tremendous impact that a thought, an image, or an emotion can have on the emotional brain, which in turn tells the body how to respond. Positive stress, such as the stress of competition when you feel confident in your ability, contributes to heightened functioning and peak performance. But bad stress, such as chronic anxiety, frequent hostility, or feeling helpless, makes you more vulnerable to negative life events such as job loss, personal injury, and trauma, which in turn generate even more stress.

For example, Jack, a corporate project manager, accepted nothing less than perfection, which led him to fret over minute details and to frequently change his mind about the course of action. Consequently, he missed deadlines and went over budget, which concerned management. Worse, Jack became known as a difficult person to work with, and employees tried to avoid his projects. His annual review was negative, citing cost overruns, missed deadlines, and low employee morale.

His department manager said he got stuck in sidetracks and could not see the "big picture." Knowing he was on thin ice, Jack worked even harder to avoid mistakes. Eventually he developed stomach problems that were so serious he had to take a leave of absence.

Unrelenting anxiety like Jack's compromises immune functioning and puts excessive demand on the cardiovascular system. Worrywarting, like what Jack was doing at work, with its parading images of disaster, keeps you in a continuous state of alarm, which wears out the body and lowers resistance to disease. Additionally, when the emotional brain responds to worry thoughts by triggering the "fight-flight" response and you do not fight or flee, but restrain yourself instead, the emotional brain interprets your immobility as insufficient preparation for the imagined disaster and increases your tension. Maintaining a high degree of alertness without relief, which is what worrywarts do, is extremely stressful and has been linked by medical research to health problems.

Anxiety Becomes a Habitual Response

You may blame a situation for causing distress, but it is actually *your response to the situation* and not the situation itself that causes the anxiety. One person's stressor is another's challenge. Worrywarts respond to a wide range of situations by becoming anxious. They scare themselves with thoughts of disaster, so more body chemicals are released, which triggers more worry and more scary images. Going from one frightening thought to another, and feeling out of control, the worrywart worries, "What's wrong with me?" It is a vicious circle caused by responding to the situation with more worry.

Some worrywarts respond to their fears by getting both anxious and angry, like Elizabeth, who said, "I get worried about my husband when he's late getting home and imagine all kinds of accidents that could have happened, convincing myself that he's dead. I berate myself for having been irritable toward him and make promises of how appreciative I'll be if only he'll return home safely. Then, when he shows up without an apology, saying he 'forgot' to call—well, I get furious at being treated so poorly and being made to worry like that!" Elizabeth's fears, combined with feelings of rage, put her doubly in danger. Being prone to anger is a stronger predictor of dying young than are other high-risk factors such as smoking, high blood pressure, and high cholesterol.

There is hope! It is the inability to cope with stressful demands and not the intensity of the events themselves that cause health problems. Worrywarts cope by worrying. As we've seen, it's an unproductive cycle. Worry begets anxiety, anxiety begets worry, in a never-ending spiral. But you can break out of the self-perpetuating trap of worry and anxiety, by learning to worry smart.

PART 2

How to Worry
Smarter

CHAPTER 6

What Is Smart Worry?

God, give us the grace to accept with serenity the things that cannot be changed, the courage to change the things which should be changed, and the wisdom to distinguish one from the other.
—DR. REINHOLD NIEBUHR

Worry's job is to anticipate danger before it arises and rehearse how to deal with it—sort of a mental fire drill. But the danger is that you will get caught in worrywarting. It reminds me of when I was a kid lying in bed at night frightened by shadows. Paralyzed, I would stare into the dark, not daring to blink and unable to go to sleep. As long as I kept my eyes on "it," I'd have a chance because I could see it coming and do something to get away or to fight "it" off. Much in the same way, worrywarts keep their mind's eye on the foreboding source of anxiety, while ignoring everything else. Smart worriers, on the other hand, catch themselves worrywarting and redirect its momentum into productive action.

Cheryl, owner of a small toy company, is an example. "When we introduced our new line of 'love bears' our distributor insisted on a run of fifty thousand units. No sooner did they hit the warehouse than sales took a nosedive. I was swamped with worrying, convinced we would never get our money back. I imagined my house in foreclosure and me becoming a bag lady. Suddenly I saw what I was doing and said to myself, 'Stop it! You're anxious, that's all. It's to be expected with so much money on the line.' Then I asked myself, 'What would a supportive friend advise me to do?' The answer was easy. 'Get out there and market those love bears.' And I thought, 'Yes! I can make sales happen. This is a challenge!' After only two calls that afternoon I got a new account and sold 1,000 units!" Cheryl stopped her worrywarting and channeled her anxiety into making sales.

The stress of having unsold love bears created vague feelings of anxiety for Cheryl, which triggered her fears of being a homeless bag lady. Had she been unable to recognize her anxious feelings she would have been at their mercy as she reacted to them.

Smart worriers don't automatically flip into worrying, like a knee-jerk reaction. Through reading their emotions, they avoid being swept away by a torrent of worry. Cheryl identified she was anxious and realized it was a natural response to financial risk—there was no imminent danger. She countered her worrisome thinking and brought herself back to balance. By worrying smart Cheryl was able to focus on solving the problem of selling an overstock of love bears. It was a problem she could solve.

Smart Worriers Soothe Themselves

The ability to soothe yourself enables you to overcome barriers and bounce back from almost any situation. Smart worriers avoid becoming consumed by the anxiety generated by studying the perils associated with a worrisome situation, by recognizing their distress as anxiety and bringing themselves back to balance. Worrywarts do the opposite. They keep themselves in a state of agitation and worry themselves sick. Smart worriers soothe themselves, while worrywarts rile themselves up.

Smart Worriers Talk to Themselves the Way a Friend Would

Worry is an inner dialogue called "self-talk," a talking it over with yourself as a way to cope with bothersome situations. This dialogue is tremendously powerful in how you feel and in shaping what you do. Worrywarts' self-talk is judgmental, critical, and scary, keeping them off-balance and unnerved as it triggers more worry.

Smart worriers talk to themselves the way a friend would. Friends encourage, give permission, and challenge extremes. For example, Cheryl, who imagined ruin because of a slowdown in love bear sales, worried smart when she talked to herself the way a friend would. By doing so she redirected her attention to finding a solution, instead of worrywarting and getting fixated on her fears.

Smart Worriers Are Hopeful

Smart worriers come away from a worry session feeling hopeful; worrywarts, on the other hand, convince themselves a situation is hopeless. Hope is a belief that success is possible, even if difficult—there is a way to get what you want. Hopeful thinking is an acquired style, a way of looking at the world that builds resiliency. With hope, you can resist anxiety and avoid defeatist attitudes that cause depression in the face of setbacks. Smart worriers think in helpful ways, which promotes hopeful feelings whereas worrywart thinking is critical and scary, triggering fear and anxiety.

Smart Worriers Think Flexibly

Philosopher Alan Watts once cautioned that problems that remain persistently insoluble should always be suspected as questions asked in the wrong way. Stuck in "rut thinking," worrywarts mentally replay the worrisome situation repetitively, getting nowhere; they work themselves into increasing levels of anxiety. Smart worriers, on the other hand, challenge their views of the worrisome situation, looking at it from several vantage points.

Smart Worriers Look for Solutions

Smart worriers focus on finding solutions. Like worrywarts, they examine dangers, but they don't get stuck, fixated like a terrified deer staring into the headlights of an oncoming car. Worry is not preparation; making a plan of action is. Once the risk has been studied and the work of worry is finished, smart worriers let go of worrying to look for solutions and contingency plans. Once they have a plan, smart worriers use their imagination to rehearse success, while worrywarts misuse imagination, envisioning the disasters they fear.

Smart Worriers Look for Partial Solutions

While worrywarts blow up the risks associated with worrisome situations, smart worriers break big worries into smaller pieces and proceed with small-step solutions to these more manageable subproblems.

Smart Worriers Accept What Cannot Be Changed

Smart worriers differentiate between what they can do something about and what they cannot change, while worrywarts worry uselessly about things they cannot change. When something is beyond control, smart worriers don't worry about it; if they did, they would create destructive anxiety. Instead they focus on what they can do, and act to make themselves feel better about what they can do nothing about.

You Can Worry Smarter

You, too, can become a smart worrier. Worrying smarter is not an either/or matter. It is something you get better and better at, and as you do, you handle bothersome situations more easily without letting worry run wild so you can enjoy life more. Using the techniques in this book you can transform yourself from a worrywart to a smart worrier. And in the process you'll feel better, sleep more soundly, and get more of what you want from life.

CHAPTER 7

Create a Time and Place to Worry

To every thing there is a season, and a time to every purpose under heaven.

—Ecclesiastes

Probably the worst thing about worrywarting is the way that it tends to crowd out everything else, spoiling your day and disrupting your sleep. It is smart to worry but only when you keep worry contained and focused on looking for solutions. When worry turns into obsessing, then it becomes a problem.

One way to keep worrying within bounds is to use a process psychologists call situation control to create a "worry place"—a special place where you do nothing but worry when there. It helps contain worrywarting, while developing smart worry skills. The power in doing this is that it creates an association between a situation—the worry place—and your response—worrying. When you experience a certain emotion repetitively in a particular situation, an association between the feelings you experienced and the situation where you felt them develops. Eventually, when you enter the situation you will feel an emotion that has become associated with the situation. For example, you usually feel contemplative and spiritual when in a church, boisterous at a football game, and like eating heartily at Thanksgiving dinner.

Choose a Place to Worry

Let's look at how Martha used this principle to worry smarter. At work she often worried away the afternoon and then had to take work home, leading to even more worrying about her job. Martha began roping in her wild worrying by creating a worry place. She picked a fire escape near her office. Next, she deliberately created an association between being on the fire escape and worrying by going there when she caught herself worrying. She said to herself, "I'm worrying. I'll go to my worry place to worry" and went to the fire escape to "worry" for three minutes. When she returned to her desk she acknowledged herself by saying, "Good. I left the worry outside. I can focus on my work now." For the next two weeks Martha went to the fire escape each time she caught herself worrying.

As the association between worrying and being on the fire escape strengthened, Martha began using it to contain her worrywarting by gradually restricting how often she could go to the fire escape. First, she set a limit of three times an hour, or every twenty minutes. When she caught herself worrying before twenty minutes had passed, she said to herself, "This is not the time or place to worry. I'll put this on my worry list so I can worry about it later," and made a written note of the worrisome concern on a "worry list" next to the phone. Martha acknowledged herself by saying, "I put the worry on my list to worry about later. That's good," and resumed working. As her ability to contain worrying grew, Martha gradually increased the time between visits to her worry place.

Eventually, Martha was able to go all day with only one or two visits to the fire escape. When there was a crisis or special stress, Martha never allowed herself to worry at her desk, but went to the worry place more often. By worrying only in the worry place and never at her desk, Martha created an association between worry and being on the fire escape and another association between being at her desk and working. As a result, Martha worried less and got more work done.

Schedule a Time to Worry

Martha's next step in containing her worry was to schedule a specific time for worrying. She choose the last fifteen minutes of her lunch hour because it would give her an opportunity to review her work worries when she still had time in the day to act on them. Each workday, Martha went to the fire escape after lunch, before returning to her desk for the afternoon's work.

Martha often didn't feel like worrying, but she went to the fire escape anyway. She made sure to take her worry list with her, and as soon as she began reading it she no longer had trouble worrying. The structure further enabled Martha to contain and focus her worrying. Concentrating on pent-up concerns for a few minutes after lunch helped Martha to structure her afternoons more efficiently. Leaving her worries behind in the worry place when she returned to her desk provided Martha with a sense of mastery over her worrying.

Dos and Don'ts When Creating a Worry Place and Time

Keep in mind the following guidelines when choosing a worry place and time:

■ **Set a Time.** Set a time each day to devote to worrying. Schedule it on your calendar, like you would with any important commitment.

■ **Do Nothing Else.** Keep your worry place pure. Do nothing there but worry. Don't eat. Don't listen to music. Don't talk on the phone. When in your worry place, you must worry. Engaging in other activities in your worry place contaminates it, weakening its power. The stronger the association between worrying and being in your worry place, the more powerful it becomes in containing your worry.

■ **Reduce Disturbance.** Pick a time and place when you are not likely to be bothered. Find an out-of-the-way place, like Martha's fire escape. Hang a "Do Not Disturb" sign on the door. Take the phone off the hook.

■ **Be a Little Uncomfortable.** Your worry place should be mildly uncomfortable so you feel somewhat glad to leave. For example, you might set up a chair in the basement or in the attic, because both are substantially devoid of stimulation and get boring so you get antsy to get back to other activities. The mild aversiveness retards worrying and makes getting back to your life more attractive.

▪ **Make It Accessible.** Your worry place should be accessible, a place where you can go easily. When the pressure piles on, knowing that you can retreat to your worry place quickly builds confidence that you can contain it.

▪ **Always Worry When in Your Worry Place.** When you are in your worry place, make yourself worry, whether you feel like it or not. By worrying on schedule, even when you do not feel like it, you learn to control worry. You can try out the techniques in this book in your worry place.

▪ **Keep a "Worry List."** When a worry comes to you and you are not in your worry place, capture the worry by writing it on a list, which will reassure your anxious mind that the worry will not be forgotten. Later, your worry list can serve as an agenda when you get to your worry place. You can look over your list and determine which worry should take priority. By picking and choosing among worries, you further reinforce the idea that you can control your worrying.

▪ **Go to Your Worry Place When a Worry Comes On.** During times of stress, when you feel worry overtaking you, go to your worry place. Even if you can't control the onset of worry, by taking it to your worry place, you control how and where you worry. Worrywarting is a powerful dynamic. You can't change it overnight. By going to your worry place when you are fretting, you use powerful principles of psychological conditioning to reprogram yourself.

- **Instruct Yourself.** When you catch yourself worrying, talk yourself through the steps of containing the worry. You might say, for example, "This is nonproductive worry. I'll write this on my list for worry time. Right now I will use my time to get something else done."

- **Pat Yourself on the Back Often.** Reward yourself for using your worry place. Talk to yourself the way a good friend would. Acknowledge yourself for catching yourself worrying and going to your worry place.

- **Do Something Pleasant After Worry Time.** Arrange to do things you like to do and that make you feel good *after* your worry time. Go out for a snack or call a friend on the phone after using your worry place, for example. Reward strengthens the association in your emotional brain between finishing worry and feeling good.

Smart Worry Has a Time and Place

Creating a worry place and time helps you contain your worry, so it will not spread from one anxiety to the next. Smart worriers use this powerful technique to focus on concerns that need attention, while keeping worry from running wild, stampeding through their days and nights.

CHAPTER 8

Watch How You Worry

You'd be surprised by how much you can observe by watching.

—Yogi Berra

You are probably impatient to do something about your worrywarting. Don't make the mistake of trying to change your worrying before you understand it. Get to know your worry first. Spiritual philosopher de Ropp, author of *The Master Game*, says we are all puppets controlled by external forces. To make the puppet dance you must understand what makes it move. By watching the puppet you can figure out when and how it moves, and then you can make the puppet do what you wish by "pulling your own strings."

The first step to worrying smarter is recognizing anxiety and getting to know when and how you worry. The tool for watching your worry is self-observation, which is stepping back from experience to watch it as you live it. The object is to study your worry behavior dispassionately, the way a scientist would, rather than becoming engulfed by the worries of the moment.

Keep a Worry Journal

To get the full benefit of watching your worry, keep a record of what you observe. Record in a diary or journal what you see when you watch yourself worrying. Add notes about your feelings at the time. Just the simple act of recording self-observations engenders a sense of control—which is vital to worrywarts who feel controlled by runaway worry. As you accumulate self-observations, review them to discover patterns in your worry, which are the strings to the puppet. You might discover, for example, that certain worries intensify after talking with your mother on the phone. Or you may see that a particular sensation in your stomach signals a worry bout. Write down these important observations, as they can help you better understand your worry behavior.

Your journal can be a spiral notebook or a blank book. A loose-leaf binder also works well because you can add and rearrange pages. You might experiment with a small notebook that you can carry in your purse or jacket pocket so that it is readily available to jot down thoughts and observations anywhere you might be. Later, during worry time, you can transfer your notes into your journal.

Let Yourself Worry

To get to know how you worry, let yourself worry so that you can study what you do when you worry. *Don't try to stop the worry.* Instead, recognize that you are worrying and focus your attention onto *watching* your thoughts—what are you telling yourself about the worrisome situation? Listen closely to the words you use. Don't edit. Record in your journal the way you talk to yourself about your worry, such as, "I told myself that they would reject me if I made a mistake." Notice your emotions and describe your feelings, such as, "I feel apprehensive." Notice and describe physical sensations, such as, "I feel my heart beating faster than normal."

Rate the Worry's Strength

Rating anxiety levels helps differentiate worries. Imagine a scale from 1 to 9, with 1 being very relaxed and 9 being very anxious. As you observe yourself worrying about a particular worrisome situation, rate your anxiety level. Remember, don't try to stop or change the worry in any way. Record the anxiety rating in your journal.

Rating the degree of anxiety you're experiencing helps you realize that not all worry has the same degree of strength. Worry is not an all-or-nothing situation, as worrywarts tend to believe. It also gives you a basis for comparison. You know whether you are getting less or more anxious and whether things are getting better or worse, for example.

Identify Worry Triggers

Usually there is something that sets you to worrying. It might be a fleeting thought or a particular feeling. Through self-observation you can pinpoint what starts your worrying. When you know what triggers your worry, you gain control and can better contain it.

The challenge is to catch a worry as near to its beginning stages as possible, preferably as soon as you experience a fleeting distressing thought. In your journal, write the worrisome thought down as close to verbatim as you can. Then write "possible worry trigger" and describe *what happened just before the thought* to uncover the worry trigger. Include your thoughts and feelings along with people and events around you. For example, talking to your mother on the phone might trigger worry about making enough money and being successful in your career. In another situation, you may discover that certain sensations in your body may trigger worrying about having a heart attack.

Watch All Kinds of Worry

Study mild, moderate, and severe worry sessions. Record in your journal what worry feels like—specifically, which sensations. Describe the setting and the worrisome situations. By getting to know how you worry and what it feels like, you are taking an important step toward becoming a smart worrier.

Use Your Worry Journal

Use your journal when trying out a technique for soothing yourself and worrying smarter. Make notes on what worked for you. Write down ideas you have for becoming a smarter worrier and suggestions other people offer.

Keep worry lists in your journal. Your journal is a good place to make notes on insights on becoming a smart worrier that you may get while reading and thinking about your way of worrywarting. You might add inspirational quotes you come across that speak to your concerns, for example. If you feel uncomfortable with writing in your journal, start with lists. Keep lists of all kinds. Describe a worry, then list all the fears hiding in it. Keep lists of your joys, those priceless moments of just feeling good. Begin by listing your pleasures and positive experiences. People who regularly list pleasures of the day report that doing so puts them into a positive frame of mind. Sometimes the effect can be almost instantaneous.

Your journal is a good place to rehearse encounters. Writing out what you will say, along with various contingencies, is a kind of reprogramming, where you write a new pattern to follow.

Use Your Journal to Release Worry

Worry often springs from feeling powerless to deal with certain stressful situations. Writing out a perplexing worry in your journal is a way to take immediate action. You gain a sense of control as you write out your worry. With pen in hand you can pull the worry apart, think it through, and if it gets to be too much, set it aside to come back to later when you are better able to focus on problem identification and finding solutions.

Evaluate Your Progress

Rating your anxiety levels provides a way to measure progress in becoming a smarter worrier and determining the effectiveness of various techniques you try. Using the anxiety scale described earlier, rate your anxiety level at the beginning of each worry session and before trying out a smart worry technique. Rate your anxiety level again at the end of the session and after the technique. Record the ratings in your worry journal along with any insights you may have. When the second rating is lower, the technique has had the desired effect. Scientists call this "pre- and posttesting" and use it to evaluate how well an intervention they are studying works.

Watch as You Become a Smarter Worrier

Getting to know how you worry is an important prerequisite to becoming a smart worrier. Don't try to stop worrying—you won't succeed. When you understand when and how you worry, you learn how to control yourself so that you can pull your own strings to worry smarter while soothing yourself.

CHAPTER 9

Talk to Yourself the Way a Friend Would

If I have lost every other friend on earth, I shall at least have one friend left, and that friend shall be down inside me.

—ABRAHAM LINCOLN

You live with an ever-present companion—you! You spend more time with yourself than with anyone else. In fact, you spend *all* your time with yourself. This internal companion talks to you continuously, virtually nonstop—even when you're sleeping! As a consequence you have more influence over yourself and more ability to create your future than anyone else. This internal companion is you talking to you inside your mind. You are the creator of your internal environment. You guide yourself, criticize yourself, give to or withhold from yourself, belittle or support yourself. The internal you feels like a distinctly different person speaking to you, but it is really you inside talking to you. How you react to a worrisome situation is largely determined by what you tell yourself about it. Through this internal dialogue you make decisions; set goals; feel happy or sad, relaxed or anxious, hopeful or lost.

Worrywarts Talk to Themselves in Anxious Ways

Worrywarts talk to themselves in ways that leave them feeling anxious, afraid, and inadequate. They talk to themselves in ways that fuddy-duddies and fussbudgets talk, magnifying trivial mistakes, making a big fuss needlessly over picayune problems. Worrywarts have selective vision; they focus on "FUD"—*F*ear, *U*ncertainty, and *D*oubt—in virtually every situation, keeping themselves in a constant state of anxiety and dread. Their fuddy self-talk creates a psychological environment that is toxic and taxing.

Smart worriers actively soothe themselves when they feel anxious, depressed, or annoyed, which enables them to bounce back quickly from disappointments and setbacks. Their self-talk creates a psychological environment that is supportive and hopeful.

The way that you talk to yourself traps you in worrywarting. To break out you must stop talking to yourself in ways that make you feel anxious, small, and helpless and start being supportive and encouraging in your self-talk. Psychologists call self-talk that is soothing and brings you back to balance "compassionate self-talk" and "the language of self-support."

Talking to yourself compassionately can be learned. Like learning any new language, learning the language of self-support takes time, practice, and dedication. Self-nurturing is not that hard, really. The key is to imagine how a good friend would talk to you. Then talk to yourself that way. The hard part is breaking fuddy self-talk habits and actually starting to talk to yourself in a compassionate and self-supportive way.

Imagine What a Friend Would Say

Think of a worry you've been dwelling on lately. For this practice, pick an easy worry, not something that is terribly distressing, just something that has been mildly nagging. For a few moments, listen to how you talk to yourself about this worry. Concentrate on what you say about the worrisome situation and how you say it. Notice the exact words you use. Write the worry out in your journal just the way you tell it to yourself. Label this "fuddy talk."

Imagine telling this worry to a dear friend. What would that friend say to be supportive and encouraging? What would your friend say to soothe you and bring you back to balance? Pay attention to the words you imagine your friend would use and how he or she would say them. Write down what your friend would say in your journal. Label this "friendly talk."

How does the way you imagine a friend would talk to you about the worry compare with how you actually talk to yourself about the worry? If you are like most worrywarts you have a double standard—one for friends and one for yourself. The way you talked to yourself was probably harsh, judgmental, and critical. You probably focused on the dire aspects of the worrisome situation and questioned your ability to handle it. How did you talk to yourself when you imagined you were a friend talking to you about the worrisome situation? You were probably comforting and supportive when talking to yourself the way a friend would. You probably soothed yourself by telling you that things are not as bad as you make them out to be and pointing out how you have the ability to meet this challenge.

Switch from Fuddy to Friendly Self-Talk

Try this. Return to the worry you used in the earlier exercise and think about it as you normally do. When you hear the fuddy self-talk say, "STOP!" very loudly inside your head and imagine seeing a stop sign in your mind. Then immediately switch to friendly self-talk and say the supportive statement you wrote in your journal.

Expect fuddy talk to sneak back in. Don't berate yourself for slipping. Instead, when it does, yell, "Stop!" and imagine the stop sign again, then *immediately switch* to friendly talk again. The fuddy talk will come back again and again. That's the way the mind works. Each time it does, yell, "Stop!" silently to yourself, imagine the stop sign, and pull yourself back to friendly talk.

The Mind Is like a Wild Elephant

The Seeker and Shaman Woman were reviewing the events of the day. "I know that worrying makes my life hell, Shaman Woman," said the Seeker. "But why can I not control my mind?"

"Your mind is like a wild elephant that you must master," said the Shaman as she handed the Seeker his tea. *"When you chain the elephant it flaps its ears, slaps its tail, and runs away."*

"That's just what my mind does. It runs wild whenever I try to control it," the Seeker said excitedly. *"What should I do when it runs away, Shaman Woman?"*

"Don't scold the elephant for running," answered the Shaman. *"Simply grab the chain and pull it back. Again and again the elephant will run away—and again and again you must pull it back. Eventually, the elephant will be tamed when it learns that you are the master."*

"Then will my wild mind obey me?" the Seeker asked.

"Then you will have great power," the Shaman replied, *"because, once tamed, both elephants and minds will work for you."*

It takes a long time to master your wild mind, especially if it is used to running on, out of control. Don't get angry at yourself for running back to the worry. Be patient with your wild mind as you firmly pull your attention back to friendly talk.

Be Supportive and Encouraging

Worrywarts fuss over what's wrong and what's missing. There is always something to worry about because you can always find fault with something, no matter how good it is. Constant criticism is demotivating and beats you down. Sadly, this is just what worrywarts do to themselves with their fuddy self-talk; they punish and hurt themselves.

A supportive friend focuses on the positive and what's working. A friend builds you up by pointing out progress and what you've done right, which fosters optimism and positive feelings. Talk to yourself the way a friend would. Use friendly self-talk to give yourself credit for steps you have taken to become a smart worrier. Avoid judging your progress or the degree of your efforts—that's fuddy self-talk. Instead, praise your efforts and improvement, even when they are small. Give yourself credit and encourage yourself with friendly self-talk. Develop a habit of actively challenging worrisome thoughts and assume a critical stance toward their assumptions in a friendly way. Remind yourself that you are a valuable and lovable person even if you don't do everything perfectly.

Practice Friendly Self-Talk

There will always be difficulties, potential for accidents, and risk of failure. How you think about life's perils is really the point of impact. *You can learn another way to think*—another way of talking to yourself. The way to begin this process of transforming yourself into a smart worrier is by catching when you talk to yourself in a fuddy way and countering those negative, irrational, and illogical views with friendly talk.

You Can Learn to Talk More Friendly to Yourself

You can break free of worrywarting and learn to worry smart. You are not sick and there is nothing to get over. It's just a matter of learning another way to talk to yourself. You will always have vexing problems and you will always feel a certain degree of anxiety about them. Worrywarting is a bad habit—one that took years to learn. Change will not take place spontaneously. It will take time and effort to learn to talk in a friendly way to yourself. Don't be so demanding and hard on yourself. Talk to yourself the way a supportive friend would.

Be patient with yourself because it takes many weeks, months, even years to refute your fuddy self-talk. Over many years you've evolved a personal mythology that governs your perceptions, your feelings, and your actions. But it is a mythology—a belief system. The way you talk to yourself is a kind of ongoing self-indoctrination. Replacing the fuddy self-talk with friendly self-talk feels uncomfortable at first—just the way any new behavior does when you're breaking an entrenched habit. The irony is that most of the time the friendly self-talk is far more accurate than is the worry. Yet, you've listened to the fuddy thinking so long that it seems true because it is so familiar. But fuddy thinking and worrywarting are self-limiting mental habits—habits you can change.

CHAPTER 10

Practice Flexible Thinking

Optimism: A cheerful frame of mind that enables a tea kettle to sing though in hot water up to its nose.

—Anonymous

Worrywarting is a habitual style of critical thinking that has become a rut. It's important to be able to look at the downside of any situation and take an accurate inventory of its faults and flaws so that they can be addressed. It's valuable to be able to foresee problems that might come up so that they can be prevented or dealt with effectively.

But critical thinking isn't useful all by itself. To be able to constructively address a problem, you need to be able to think about what the solutions might be. And it's no use to anticipate problems unless you can think creatively about what you're going to do when they come up. In other words, the kind of thinking that characterizes worrywarting doesn't do you any good unless you can balance it with *other kinds of thinking*. Just as healthy eating calls for a balanced meal drawing from a variety of food groups, healthy coping requires a balance of different thinking styles.

Styles of thinking can also be compared to tools in a tool kit. The worrywart is like a carpenter who has boxes and boxes of nails but has forgotten she also has a hammer in her toolbox. Without the hammer, all the nails in the world won't do her any good; they just become a huge collection of sharp, pointed objects that can scratch, pierce, and scrape when handled, just as the worrywart's endless negative critical thoughts become abrasive to her peace of mind.

Habits die hard. Behavioral psychologists say that it's much easier to get rid of a bad habit by replacing it with another habit than to try to quit doing something that you're accustomed to doing without putting anything in its place.

You can replace the bad habit of fuddy self-talk with its critical thinking, with the good habit of feeding your peace of mind with a balanced diet of basic thinking styles that, when used together, provide a constructive mental approach to any worrisome situation you have to think about.

Six Thinking Styles

Creativity expert Edward DeBono identified six basic styles of thinking: objective, emotive, supportive, possibility, critical, and strategic. For each style of thinking there is a corresponding question. Asking yourself this question will automatically set the corresponding thinking style in motion.

Objective Thinking
Ask yourself: "What are the facts?"

The cool-headed, no-nonsense manner of Sergeant Friday in the popular 1950s TV show "Dragnet" epitomizes objective thinking. When interviewing witnesses who were getting emotional or opinionated about a crime, Sergeant Friday would try to get them back on track with his famous line, "Just the facts, ma'am."

The key to objective thinking is to separate emotions, opinions, reactions, desires, and preconceptions from the plain facts of a situation. For instance, it may be a *fact* that your boss or neighbor did something that makes you angry. In this case, it is also a *fact* that you are angry. However, no matter how obvious it may seem to you that this person is a jerk, this is not really a fact. It *is* a fact, however, that you *think* this person is a jerk.

Worrywarts often forget to separate facts from *negative possibilities*. For instance, if a worrywart's teenage son has borrowed the family car and failed to return home when expected, it may not even occur to the mother that anything short of a catastrophe has taken place. She might make a panicked phone call to a friend and report, "Something horrible has happened!" just as if this were fact. The only *facts* of the situation, however, are that the kid has not returned home and has not called. It's far more likely that the son has gotten caught up with having fun with his friends—such a harmless possibility may not even cross the worried mother's mind.

Practicing objective thinking helps bring you back to balance because it reminds you that the facts of a situation are not the same as the disastrous scenarios you envision when worrywarting. Furthermore, separating out the facts of a situation through objective thinking is a prerequisite for formulating a sound plan of action based on realistic possibilities. Knowing that the plan you choose is based on an assessment of actual facts will help to inspire confidence in your decision while decreasing unnecessary worry.

Emotive Thinking
Ask yourself: "What am I feeling?"

To see the facts of a situation clearly you must accurately identify emotions so that their presence doesn't cloud the facts. Practicing emotional thinking—answering the question "What am I feeling?"—will help prevent your ideas, actions, and decisions from being driven by your emotions in ways of which you are not aware.

Emotions are often contradictory and seemingly irrational. However, we tend to think that our feelings have to be "justified." If you put pressure on yourself to have only emotions that "make sense," you may end up unconsciously distorting your assessment of a situation to fit your emotions, or you may fail to acknowledge your true feelings because they don't fit the situation. For instance, you may believe that you shouldn't be angry at someone unless they've done something that "deserves" exactly the amount of anger you feel. If so, you might blow out of proportion the severity of an incident that angered you a great deal or, alternatively, fail to recognize how angry you really are. But the fact is, you're still just as angry as you are whether or not you think you "should" be. So, when you engage in emotive thinking, consider *all* of your feelings about the situation in question, whether or not they seem justified, whether or not they make sense, and even if they contradict each other.

Physical sensations can be linked to emotions, so include physical sensations such as butterflies in the stomach, which can be a manifestation of anxiety, or a lump in the throat, which could indicate that you are sad about something.

Worry and anxiety are often a response to fear that a desired result will not be forthcoming or that a very *undesirable* result may be on the way. When performing emotive thinking, also bring into consideration your preferences, likes and dislikes, values, and desires, which are ways of looking at what you want—and don't want—out of a situation.

When the worried mother, whose teenage son was late returning home with the car, engaged emotive thinking, she realized that she was afraid that something untoward had happened to her son. She also realized that she was angry that he was late returning home with the car and hadn't called her to let her know what was going on. Finally, she realized that having these feelings didn't mean that something had happened to her son.

Supportive Thinking
Ask yourself: "What's working?"

Supportive thinking looks at the positive aspects of a situation and focuses on ways to enhance them. Make a list of what's right, what's working in the worrisome situation, and detail strengths and assets of everyone involved—including yours—along with positive resources available for dealing with the situation or making it better. When the mother, worrying about her son being late getting home with the car, asked herself, "What's working?" she came up with the following supportive thinking. Her son is responsible and doesn't speed or drink. He's such a good driver that he won a teen driving contest. Finally, she thought about the fact that the car is rated as one of the safest on the road.

Supportive thinking often feels unnatural to worrywarts who tend to focus on weaknesses, what's wrong, what's not working, and what might go wrong. Engaging supportive thinking brings you back to a more balanced view of the situation.

Possibility Thinking

Ask yourself: "What's possible here?"

When engaged in possibility thinking, let your creativity run. Sometimes you have to prompt it by deliberately thinking about worrisome situations in the opposite way from how you usually would, or "turning it upside down." For instance, if a person has wronged you in some way, think of how the person is an ally and imagine how you actually benefit from the offending act. Look at weaknesses and disadvantages and try to see how they might be strengths and advantages. This is often called turning lemons into lemonade.

Brainstorm new options for handling a worrisome situation. Don't try to be logical or realistic. Entertain silly, even absurd ideas in order to uncover alternatives that you have never thought of before. The key is to allow your mind the unfettered imaginative freedom of a child at play. The difficult aspect of this, especially for the worrywart, is to avoid critiquing your ideas, dismissing them before you can see where they lead. You have to suspend your critical faculty in order to move into new territory. Even the most unrealistic or implausible scenarios often contain seeds of valuable new ideas, which in the end turn out to have practical applications.

When the worried mother employed possibility thinking, she thought of the car running out of gas and her son losing the keys. "Maybe his watch stopped." Then a silly idea crossed her mind, "Suppose he eloped!" She laughed at the thought. It opened a whole range of possibilities. "Maybe he's doing a good deed. Maybe the coach introduced him to an agent and he's trying out for an athletic scholarship!"

Critical Thinking
Ask yourself: "What's wrong or could go wrong?"

Critical thinking is where worrywarts get stuck. It is also the dominant thinking style of perfectionists—most of whom are worrywarts—who constantly focus on finding flaws in everything.

Critical thinking looks for what is wrong or could go wrong, identifies risks, and makes judgments, such as good or bad, right or wrong, black or white. Critical thinking is linear and logical—if this, then that. It's easy to get trapped in a rut of critical thinking. Having seen the flaws and imperfections in a person, thing, or situation, it's hard to forget about them long enough to perceive strong points or even facts, for that matter. This is why, when analyzing a situation, it's advisable to engage objective and supportive thinking *before* critical thinking.

Furthermore, our society encourages, teaches, and rewards critical thinking in school, where students are assigned to find flaws in an essay, argument, or research design, without necessarily discussing its strong points. Politics in our country has become so dominated by finding flaws that political campaigns focus far more on the weaknesses and liabilities of the opposing candidate than on their own candidate's qualifications, positive ideas, or past achievements. Even workbooks for small children ask, "what's *wrong* with this picture?" but never "what's right with this picture?" In fact, the English language itself has far more negative and critical nouns and adjectives than words of praise. No wonder so many of us become worrywarts!

Nonetheless, critical thinking *is* an important skill, a necessary part of a balanced diet of thinking styles. Without the ability to make an accurate assessment of the real risks in a worrisome situation, you are likely to encounter many avoidable difficulties. However, in order for critical thinking to be helpful, it must occur within the context of a full range of thinking styles.

The worried mother was well versed in critical thinking, especially in imagining what *could* go wrong. "He could be hurt!" was her first thought. Pressing herself to identify other things that could have gone wrong, she realized he could have had a flat tire, been kidnapped, gotten lost, or even run away!

Strategic Thinking
Ask yourself: "What's the next step?"

Once you've engaged each of the preceding five thinking styles, you have identified the facts of the worrisome situation;

considered how you feel about it, what you want and what you don't want to happen, and what's right and what's working; looked at it from unusual angles and surprising perspectives; and identified what's wrong and what could go wrong. The final step is to view the worrisome situation from a detached perspective, taking all the information you've gathered into account to decide which type of thinking is most appropriate in determining your next step. Do you need to focus on something that's right about the situation and take advantage of this asset? Do you need to focus on something that's seriously wrong with the situation and attempt to fix it? Do you need to pay more attention to your emotions, and to work with the situation to move toward a result that benefits you most? Or do you need to approach the situation from an entirely new angle that you hadn't considered before? Chances are your next step will be some combination of the six thinking styles.

When the worried mother reviewed the results of her previous thinking, she realized that she needed to return to supportive and possibility thinking because she had to soothe herself while she examined what actions, if any, she might take.

Practice Flexible Thinking

You can break out of habitual critical thinking by viewing a worrisome situation through the different lenses provided by the six thinking styles. This practice will dislodge you from being stuck in catastrophizing about the worrisome situation by getting you to think about it more fully.

At first it may be somewhat difficult to practice flexible thinking about a situation that is truly stressful to you because your tendency will be to go straight to critical thinking and get stuck there once again.

In the beginning, flexible thinking will be easier if you practice it on situations that are not particularly sensitive, avoiding highly charged situations. As your skill and ability at flexible thinking grow, you can then begin to use it to analyze increasingly worrisome issues.

How to Practice

Take a mildly worrisome situation and one by one ask yourself the questions used to engage the six styles of thinking. Go through the process slowly, allowing your mind to mull over each question fully, while maintaining the style of thinking you are practicing. When you slip into another kind of thinking, stop and return to the question associated with the style of thinking you were practicing when you got sidetracked. Write your answers in your journal.

Sticking to the sequence of thinking styles laid out here is important. Critical thinking is saved almost until the end of the sequence, until just before strategic thinking—in which you make a decision about your next step. Following this sequence will help to thwart the tendency to begin with critical thinking and remain there.

CHAPTER 11

Challenge the Worry

Be gone, dull care, I prithee be gone from me!
Be gone, dull care! Thou and I shall never agree.

—JOHN PLAYFORD, *The Musical Companion*

An unchallenged worrisome thought repeated over and over gains persuasive power through a kind of self-brainwashing that becomes so compelling you forget it is only one way of looking at the situation. Soon you believe the worry to be an established fact. Once you've convinced yourself of the truth of your worry, you soon find yourself caught in the vicious circle of worrywarting, where nothing is solved as you make yourself sick with worry.

There is always more than one way to view things. Challenging a worrisome thought by contemplating a range of equally plausible points of view keeps the worry from being taken as true. If you see yourself as trapped and helpless, you'll feel depressed; whereas if you look on the situation as a difficult but surmountable challenge, you're likely to feel hopeful determination. Although it doesn't seem so, it is actually a matter of choice. You can choose among ways of viewing a worrisome situation by the way you think about it.

Although you may not be able to control a worrisome event, *you can control what you say to yourself about it.* When you do, you change your view and how you feel. This is exactly what smart worriers do. Instead of giving in to worrywarting, smart worriers actively challenge worrisome thoughts.

Events themselves don't cause you to worry; it's what you tell yourself *about* the event that leads to worrywarting. If you tell yourself the event is awful, you're going to respond with anxiety. But telling yourself awful stories is only one of many ways to talk to yourself about an event. Smart worriers talk to themselves the way a supportive friend would. Friends challenge worries and one-way thinking, and offer alternative views. Friends say, "Look at it this way . . ." And that's exactly what smart worriers do—they challenge worrisome thoughts and consider other ways of looking at it.

How to Challenge Worries

Automatic thoughts—those quick comments you make to yourself that are so well practiced they pass through your mind unnoticed and unchallenged—are usually behind worrywarting. Automatic thoughts are almost always unrealistic, irrational, and distorted. They are the sparks that ignite the wildfire, setting the cycle of worry into motion.

Identify Worrisome Thoughts

The first step in challenging worries is to become consciously aware of anxiety-provoking automatic thoughts *as they occur.* Rebecca, for example, was a professional woman in her sixties and unemployed because the company where she worked for thirty-five years went out of business. She was depressed and frightened. Even though she was financially secure she worried constantly about getting a job. When Rebecca listened to the thoughts going through her mind, she discovered that thoughts like, "Useless now!" "All I've done is worth nothing," and "No one will hire me!" frequently came to mind.

When Rebecca recognizes her automatic thoughts, she can dispute them by focusing on contradicting evidence, or she can come up with a different explanation, called "retribution." Instead of letting her worries run amok, she can learn to control what she thinks and when she thinks it.

Carry a notepad in your purse or pocket so you can write down worrisome thoughts that cross your mind throughout the day. Write the thought down as soon as you can after you notice it. If you wait, you're likely to forget it. Also note the feelings you experienced when thinking the worrisome thought.

Several times a day, review the "data" you've collected. For each worrisome thought, ask yourself: "What was going on in my mind at the time?" Record your answer next to the thought.

Brainstorm Alternative Views

In your journal, write one of the worrisome thoughts you identified. Under it write in large letters: "Challenges." Switch to possibility thinking and brainstorm several alternative views of the situation. Deliberately try to escape critical thinking. Think of absurd views. Don't try to be logical. Suspend judgment—which is particularly hard for worrywarts who are quick to judge. When Rebecca became aware of her negative automatic thoughts, she began actively refuting them by saying to herself things like, "I no longer need to work. I can do what I want now. My challenge is figuring out what I enjoy doing and how to spend my time."

Ask Challenging Questions

Asking questions about the worrisome situation is a good way to challenge the worry and uncover alternative ways of talking to yourself about it. Some of the questions listed below may help you.

Challenges
What is the evidence for this?
How else can I think about this?
How would a friend view this?
What is the worst that could happen?
What are the odds of this happening?
Is it really a crisis?
Will worrying help it?

There is no *right* answer to these questions. Your objective is to look for alternative ways of thinking, a way that soothes you so that you can deal more effectively with the issue. The problem with worrywarting is getting stuck in a view that scares you.

Catch and Challenge Worries

When you are trapped in worrywarting, get out your journal. Describe your worry in detail. Then, challenge your worry with the questions listed above and write the answers in your journal. Take your time in formulating your challenges. They are important! Read over the answers to your challenges several times.

Let the worry come into your mind and think about its bothersome aspects for a few moments, then yell, "Stop!" loudly inside your head and imagine a stop sign. Then immediately switch your thoughts to the challenges you wrote in your journal. When the worry intrudes, yell, "Stop!" and picture the stop sign again and switch your attention to rebutting your worry. When in your worry place is a good time to practice catching and challenging worries.

Challenge Impossible Demands

Worrywarts hold themselves to a strict standard no one could meet. Then they worry that they will fall short. Their fuddy talk goes nonstop, pointing out failings and all the things that could go wrong. It's awfully hard to work and excel when you're constantly faced with not quite making the mark, no matter how hard you work or how much you actually achieve.

Give yourself permission to be human, the way a good friend would. Supportive friends challenge impossible demands, urging you to go easy on yourself and to set yourself up to win.

They give you permission to make mistakes, to be less than perfect. Friends believe in you and help you believe in yourself.

Give Yourself Permission to Be Less than Perfect

When you give yourself permission to be less than perfect by talking friendly to yourself, you discover a new freedom. Intellectually, you know that making mistakes is part of learning. When you give yourself permission and let go of constantly judging your errors, it begins to *feel* okay to make mistakes. Your friendly self-talk reminds you that a mistake is one step closer to a success. Equally important is giving yourself permission to have feelings and be human, without constantly worrying about how you're failing and what you are doing wrong. Following are several examples of permissive statements:

Permissive Statements
Everyone makes mistakes.
I can take my time.
I can say no.
So what if...
It's okay to look silly.
That's an unrealistic standard.
I learn from every mistake.
Making mistakes is part of learning.

Some people like to pick out one statement that has particular meaning to them and say it over and over, almost like a mantra. "Everyone makes mistakes." "Everyone makes mistakes." "Everyone makes mistakes." Or "I can take my time." "I can take my time." "I can take my time." This is particularly effective when combined with slow, deep breathing. When you frighten yourself with "What if . . . ?" statements, give yourself permission with, "So what if . . . ?"

Permissive Flash Cards

Another powerful technique is to collect a list of twenty to thirty (or more) permissive statements in your journal. Get a package of note cards and rewrite the statements from your list on to the cards, with one per card. Read the statements on the cards several times a day. You can carry the cards with you in your purse or suit pocket. Anytime you are stuck waiting, for example, pull out your cards and read a few permissive statements. Do this for several days to familiarize your demanding emotional mind with permissive statements. Add cards whenever you think of new statements.

If you are going to do something that feels good, such as take a coffee break, call a friend, or watch a favorite TV show, you can use this rewarding activity to help your emotional mind to accept your new friendly permissive self-talk. It is easy and powerful. Here's what to do: Before engaging in the rewarding activity, read one or more permissive flash cards, then "reward" yourself by calling your friend or watching the TV show. The rewarding activity works as a reinforcement, teaching your emotional mind to allow you to be less than perfect.

Smart Worriers Challenge Their Worries

Worrywarts get stuck in extreme ideas, including that they must be perfect. Smart worriers catch themselves when they catastrophize and challenge the underlying premises. They catch themselves demanding that they perform perfectly and give themselves permission to make mistakes—to be human. Challenging your worries will give you a sense of control over your worrying that is soothing and brings you back to balance.

CHAPTER 12

Look for Solutions

Become a possibilitarian. No matter how dark things seem to be or actually are, raise your sights and see the possibilities—always see them, for they're always there.

—Norman Vincent Peale

Worry is beneficial and useful provided you worry smart. Smart worry leads to action, to doing something to improve your situation. Worry that doesn't lead to action is useless, even destructive. It is worrywarting, obsessing on uncertainties and building anxiety, keeping you frozen in inaction. Smart worry pushes you to act, to look for solutions. When there is nothing you can do, it is smart to distract yourself from the worry—and that is exactly what smart worriers do.

Identify Your Worry

Worrying isn't always at the awareness level. You can be worrying and not really be aware of it. It just seems to be going on automatically while you're doing something else, such as driving the car or making dinner. You must bring the worry to your conscious attention before you can find a solution. Begin with the question, "What am I worrying about?"

When you have identified the worry, ask the second question, "Is there anything I can do about this?" If the answer to this question is no, then there is absolutely no gain, no benefit in continuing to worry about it. Such worry will not be productive—it can't be because there is nothing you can do. To continue worrying is worrywarting—obsessing. In this case the smart worrier finds a distraction to divert attention from the useless worry.

But don't be too quick to answer no to the question of your doing something about the worrisome situation. For one thing, saying no can lead to feelings of powerlessness, which damage motivation, leading to burnout and depression. The fact is, there is almost always something you can do.

If you ask the question "Is there anything I can do about this?" and you answer yes, it is a signal to look for solutions. Once again, there is no reason to continue worrying about it. The worry has been useful and done its job—it prodded you into problem solving. Smart worriers change gears, switch thinking styles to let go of the worry, and assume a problem-solving attitude.

Problem Solving

Problem solving is divided into three important steps. The first step is the one most often skipped: defining the problem. Only when you thoroughly understand the problem, its risks, its limits, and so forth, should you move to generating options and alternatives. The final step is implementing your solution.

Redefining worries as problems to solve and then looking for solutions is almost impossible to do when worrywarting.

Finding solutions requires flexible thinking, but when you're worrywarting you're stuck in a thinking rut—that's part of the destructiveness of worrywarting. Finding solutions will be easier when you can change your thinking to a way that is optimal for the problem-solving step at hand. You might go back to Chapter 10 to review the six thinking styles because they are very useful in finding solutions.

Identify the Problem

Identifying the problem is vitally important. A vague feeling of unease, of anxiety, or of depression is hard to tackle. The troublesome situation must be clearly identified and named. This is where you switch to objective thinking—fact finding. What are the facts, ma'am? Who? What? Where? When? How? After you have thoroughly reviewed all of the facts, switch to emotive thinking to explore how you feel about the worrisome situation. What is worrisome about the situation? What are your desires relative to this worry? Next, switch to supportive thinking and explore the positives of the situation. What is working? What is right about this situation? What resources do you have for dealing with it? Who are your allies? List answers to these questions in your journal.

Brainstorm Options

The next step is to generate multiple options for solving the problem. Now is the time to switch to possibility thinking where you assume a creative mind-set. Search for new approaches and alternatives. Don't rule out any idea, no matter how preposterous it may seem. In fact, it helps to actively try to think of absurd options. Not only can it help you to escape from thinking ruts, but sometimes an idea that seems silly at first turns out to be a brilliant breakthrough. Other times, crazy ideas act as stepping-stones to a new creative approach. Write all your ideas down. Don't censor any idea.

When you have identified several potential solutions, switch to critical thinking to evaluate their merits. For each possibility, ask what is bad about it. What could go wrong if you implemented this solution? What are the weaknesses of this option? Write down the identified negatives next to the potential solution. After you have done this for each potential solution, compare the solutions, weighing the possible negatives of each against the negatives of the other potential solutions.

Look for Partial Solutions

You can defeat yourself by demanding too much too soon. Smart worriers know how to set themselves up to succeed by breaking the problem into manageable pieces. One of the hardest things to do is to get started. The philosopher Kierkegaard said that it isn't a person's accomplishment that is laudable; it is that the person made a beginning. This is heroic because at the beginning you don't know if you will succeed or fail. But you must make a beginning to accomplish anything. Starting is difficult because you must overcome your inertia. One trick that makes beginning easier is to keep breaking the problem into smaller and smaller pieces until you find a piece that you can do something about now. Then do that small step and you have made a beginning!

Rita, for example, was paralyzed by worrying about the impact report she had to prepare. She just couldn't get started. So she broke the process into steps, including researching the literature, interviewing key people, preparing an outline, and so forth. The smaller steps were not as intimidating and she was able to get started on the report.

Of course, you should expect that at some point you may run out of steam so that your progress stops. This is natural and happens to all of us. Here again, the critical skill is making a beginning—starting again. Don't be so concerned about finishing something; focus on beginning, again and again, until you finally finish.

In addition to looking for partial solutions, think in terms of "almost" perfect. Work on something, then improve it bit by bit. Avoid *shoulds* and other demands to do everything all at once, immediately and perfectly. Set yourself up to succeed by looking for almost perfect, partial solutions.

Trying Out Solutions

From your brainstorming, select a solution to try out. A good place to try out potential solutions is in your imagination.

Your imagination is like a theater where you can test solutions and practice new approaches.

The technique is simple but powerful. First, take several slow, deep breaths to relax yourself. Imagine that your mind is a stage where you set the props, you have any actors you choose, and you are the director. The idea is to enact the solution you are considering on your mental stage while imagining what would happen. Pay close attention to your emotions during the imaginary enactment. How you feel is important information. Notice how other people respond, and imagine how they feel. Study this drama on your mental stage as dispassionately and objectively as you can. Switch to strategic thinking to decide how to proceed. You might want to alter the proposed solution or enact it differently. Try these modifications out on your stage.

Ben, for example, is an engineer who was promoted to manager. He soon learned he hated being a supervisor. He was depressed, and it was threatening his performance and his relationship with his wife. He contemplated asking to be relieved of his management duties and to be reassigned to project development, which he loved doing. To prepare, he imagined working on decoding projects and noticed an immediate improvement in his mood, which confirmed that leaving management was the right thing to do. But then he worried about how his wife, boss, and co-workers would react. One by one Ben role-played on his mental stage, breaking the news to these significant others in his life. He imagined what he would say and tried out several replies until he found those that worked best.

Using a journal in conjunction with practicing on your mental stage will help you work through this exercise. Record impressions after trying out a solution. Describe your feelings. Describe how others felt when you imagined being them. What was the outcome? The journal technique is especially useful when you don't have someone you trust to talk the worrisome situation and possible solutions over with.

When you shape a solution that feels right in your imagination, it is time to try it out in real life. If you are at all anxious about carrying out the solution, then it is a good idea to rehearse it on your mental stage many times. When rehearsing you should breathe deeply and slowly to keep relaxed. *It is important to imagine the solution working for you and your feeling better afterward.*

Try out the solution and evaluate what happens. What worked? What could have been improved? Remember to look for partial success. Keep repeating the process of imagining solutions, rehearsing them mentally, carrying them out, then evaluating what happens. Continue in this process of translating the worry into a problem to solve and then trying out partial solutions. Persistence is important. Continue until you feel better.

Keep notes in your journal so you can remember insights you've gotten while doing this. Keeping a journal facilitates your efforts at self-change because it gives you a way to review what you have learned as well as a way to see your progress. Seeing progress promotes success.

When you worry smart and look for solutions, you feel better because you get your mind off your fear and onto action. You gain perspective, feel in command, and return to balance.

CHAPTER 13

Set Worries Aside

> *He who takes to himself a joy*
> *Doth the winged life destroy,*
> *But he who kisses the joy as it flies*
> *Lives in eternity's sunrise.*

—William Blake

Worrywarts become so fixated on worrisome issues that they can't stop thinking about them. You just can't let go! You cling to a worry, repeating it continuously in your mind, as if you're afraid you'll forget it. Worrywarts will worry all evening long, spoiling what could have been a pleasant break. This obsessiveness locks you into a constant battle against vague feelings of distress, which becomes an ongoing drain on your vitality, undermining your ability both to deal effectively with the source of the worry and to enjoy yourself.

Smart worriers soothe themselves by setting aside worries when they arise. It's natural and inevitable that concerns of your life will pop into your mind periodically. The trick is to prevent yourself from becoming fixated in worry every time this happens. This can be accomplished by cultivating an attitude of *detached concern.*

Detached Concern

An attitude of detached concern short-circuits the cycle of worrywarting, in which a worry stimulates anxiety that breeds more worry, which breeds more anxiety. However, since the tendency to fixate on worrisome thoughts is so entrenched in most of us, especially worrywarts, the ability to set such thoughts aside must be learned.

Detached concern can be likened to the way in which a mirror reflects images. As long as you stand in front of a mirror, it reflects your image. As soon as you move away from the mirror, however, it no longer reflects your image and reflects the image of whatever is now directly before it instead. The mirror does not hold on to or cling to the image of any object even for the briefest instant after that object has moved away from the mirror; rather, the mirror lets go of the image immediately. Conversely, a mirror accepts all objects that are placed before it, reflecting their images as long as they are in front of it. A mirror does not reject an object by refusing to reflect its image.

Detached concern has a similar relationship to thoughts. This mental attitude accepts all thoughts, fighting none of them, but lets go of them quickly as well. Treat your thoughts the way the mirror treats images—accepting and letting go.

Detached concern allows you to set aside intrusive thoughts. It's important not to confuse setting thoughts aside with fighting, resisting, or forcefully trying to make them go away. Engaging your worrisome thoughts in this kind of battle saps energy. Either way, you get stuck obsessively thinking about the worrisome situation.

Leave Worry on the Side of the Road

The Shaman Woman and the Seeker were practicing a quiet meditation while walking along a muddy road. They came to a strange man wearing fancy shoes, calling to a little dog on the other side of the road.

When the Seeker and the Shaman Woman came near, the man said to the Shaman, "My little dog cannot hear me when I call, and if I cross this muddy road to get him, I will ruin my fancy shoes! Woman, will you get my dog from across the road?"

Without speaking or even breaking her stride, the Shaman Woman stepped to the other side of the road, lifted the little dog into her arms, crossed the muddy road, and set the dog down next to the man with the fancy shoes. Then she continued walking in silence.

Later, when they had reached their destination and completed the meditation, the Seeker, who was agitated, said, "Shaman Woman, why did you stop to help that man with his dog? You know that strange dogs can be dangerous. It could have bitten you! It might have had rabies! And the man could have been up to some kind of trick! He might have been a robber—or worse! Why were you so reckless?"

The Shaman Woman replied, "I left the little dog on the side of the road. Are you still carrying it?"

The words *detached* and *concern* seem to contradict each other. It's normal to become somewhat attached to, or fixated on, issues that you're concerned about. However, while you can't stop caring about issues important to you—nor would you want to—you can cultivate distanced objectivity characterized by decreased emotional intensity.

Here's how Marlene practiced detached concern one rainy day. It was starting to rain when Marlene left work for the long, tedious drive home. She remembered that she left her treasured quilt out on the deck to air out. It was getting wet in the rain! "'Oh, no!' was my first response as I speeded up. Then I realized that driving faster wouldn't help and might cause an accident. I thought of what I could do to repair the wet quilt. Then I said to myself, 'I have a plan. There's no more I can do now. Just let it go! Leave it on the side of the road.' Each time I fell back into the worry about the quilt, I repeated, 'Let it go!' It helped and I was able to drive more cautiously and enjoy the rainbow over the Bay."

The Relaxation Response

The term "relaxation response" was coined by Herbert Benson, M.D., who popularized it in his well-known book of the same name. The physiology of the relaxation response involves an increase in slow brain-wave activity; slowing of metabolism, heart rate, and breathing; and lowering of blood pressure. Through his research, Benson has observed that "repeated activation of the relaxation response [can] mend the internal wear and tear brought on by stress." When the relaxation response is triggered, says Benson, "your mind and body suddenly become a five-star resort in which all the service personnel make your restoration and health their priority and are especially concerned with alleviating the harmful effects of stress. . . . [A] great team of stress-busters and body relaxers emerges when everyday thoughts and worries are put aside."

The relaxation response is a natural physiological mechanism that tends to return both the body and the mind to a state of balance. Cultivating the relaxation response initiates a *cycle of soothing* that is the antidote to the cycle of worry, fixation, and anxiety so familiar to worrywarts. As you begin to evoke the tranquility of the relaxation response regularly, worrisome thoughts will tend to arise less frequently, and it will be easier to release them when they do. As a result, your overall level of anxiety will decrease over time with the practice of the relaxation response.

How to Elicit the Relaxation Response

According to Benson, there are only two steps that must be followed to elicit the relaxation response. First, repeat a word, sound, prayer, phrase, or muscular activity. Then, passively disregard intrusive thoughts that come to mind, and return to your repetition.

Repetition of a word or activity is the key to letting go of intrusive, worrisome thoughts, preventing your mind from fixating on them by providing a soothing *alternative focus* for your mental attention. When a worrisome thought intrudes, passively disregard it and return your attention to the word or activity you are repeating.

Benson recommends practicing the relaxation response for two twenty-minute sessions every day. He says that "the relaxation response can be evoked by any of a large number of techniques, including certain types of prayer . . . progressive muscular relaxation, jogging, swimming, Lamaze breathing exercises, yoga, tai chi chuan, chi gong, and even knitting and crocheting."

Part 3 of this book presents a variety of simple ways to soothe yourself and worry smarter. Several of these techniques soothe by eliciting the relaxation response, including breathing deeply while counting inhales and exhales, rocking yourself, taking a warm bath, releasing muscle tension, and counting worry beads. With other techniques, promoting the relaxation response is secondary to other smart-worry benefits, including distracting yourself by counting things, smiling and laughing, saying a little prayer, and all kinds of physical exercise.

In your journal keep notes about your experiences. Remember to rate your anxiety level before and after using the soothing technique. Describe what worked, how you felt doing the exercise, and any thoughts and insights you might have.

Decompress Tension and Anxiety

Many worrywarts bring work worries home so that even though they may be home or at a movie with friends, their minds are still working away. A lot of people use alcohol to decompress.

They may make a ritual of going to the local "watering hole" for a couple of beers after work, for example. Others smoke a joint or take a Valium as soon as they get home. While an occasional drink with friends after work is not a problem, it's advisable to avoid using alcohol or drugs to decompress because the potential for addiction is just too high. If you find that you are habitually using alcohol or drugs to soothe yourself, it is a good idea to seek information and support for breaking this dangerous habit. You might talk with your personal physician or clergy, who may refer you to a beneficial program. Alternatively, talking with a good friend can be helpful. It is difficult to break free of worrywarting if you are simultaneously struggling with an addiction.

A simple technique called decompression can be used to create a release from pressure and to unwind from work. Decompression is a planned, routine behavior you use to create a relaxing routine to mark the end of your workday so that you can unwind and make the transition to personal time.

Engage in a Pleasant Routine

The key factor in decompression is the routine. Routine creates structure and marks the time of the day. Walking the dog is a good example. Ann, a writer working out of her home, walks her little dog, Sir William, every evening at 5:00 P.M.—rain or shine. Walking Willie denotes the end of working and the beginning of evening. Routine helps other people honor her boundaries, as well. Ann's friends know to wait until she gets home to phone or visit.

The idea behind decompression is to deliberately train yourself in a helpful habitual routine. The essential idea is to create an association between being in the situation and a particular activity and mood. As the routine becomes a *routine* you will find yourself *feeling* like doing it. Then when you engage in the routine it triggers soothing feelings. Returning to the example with Ann, who has been walking Willie every evening for more than four years, this decompression routine has become a trigger for unwinding from the pressure of writing and turning her mental focus to evening social activities.

Developing a routine is a form of conditioning, and that's why breaking a routine is so difficult—because you're conditioned to feel and act in certain ways. Usually you're not aware of learning routines until you've become entrenched in these habits. Developing a routine is difficult when you're just starting. You must be very deliberate in establishing the activities of your decompression routine.

Pick an Enjoyable Activity

The decompression activity can be anything you find enjoyable and gets your mind off your job. Reading, engaging in hobbies, and doing things with friends or family are popular. Or, if you've been with people all day, it may be relaxing to do something alone. George, for example, loves to cook. For him, stopping at his local green grocer to select the freshest vegetables for dinner is a good way to unwind. He doesn't rush through shopping. Instead, he thinks of it as an end in itself. He takes time to savor the smell of fennel in the vegetable aisle. He enjoys the perfect beauty of a ripe apple. When George arrives home, he is relaxed and refreshed. As another example, Jeffrey, who lives a half block from a small pond, takes a half hour each day, except in bad weather, to walk down to the pond with day-old bread to feed the ducks.

Exercise Is Good for Decompressing

An exercise routine is a natural decompresser. Just by getting your muscles into motion, you release tension and burn fat. When you exercise you release muscle tension, while your brain manufactures soothing endorphins that act like a natural opiate. Exercising on the way home from work can have very beneficial returns. Leslie combined a clothes-changing routine with exercise. At the end of each day, she changes from her high-heeled shoes into running shoes before beginning her two-mile jog home.

Establishing an exercise routine takes discipline. Make it easy for yourself. Find a gym somewhere along your route home so that you don't have to go out of your way. Be creative! Rent a locker where you can keep a change of clothes, for example. Then you can shower after your workout and step right into your evening outfit, ready for a dinner date, a night at the movies, or time with the kids. If you're worried in the morning, you can stop off at the gym to work it off. In fact, morning exercise is a great routine for starting your day off right.

Let Worries Go

Worrywarts cling to their worries, which go around and around in their heads, stressing them out and diminishing their quality of life. Smart worriers, on the other hand, use the relaxation response, decompression, and other techniques to leave worries on the side of the road. They soothe themselves in the process so that they can get on with living the good life.

CHAPTER 14

Imagine Positive Possibilities

> *Some men see things as they are and say, why; I*
> *dream things that never were and say, why not.*
>
> —Robert F. Kennedy

When you imagine terrible things that might happen, your emotional mind responds as if the dreaded events are real and actually happening. When you fret over things you must do next week, for example, your emotional mind responds as if the bothersome situation were happening now. To the emotional mind it is always "now"; there is no past or future and there is no distinction between real and imagined. This poses a problem for worrywarts whose imaginations are filled with awful pictures of negative possibilities.

Your Body Thinks What You Imagine Is Real

A paralyzing imagination can be retooled to help you become a smarter worrier. To better understand the power of imagination, try the following experiment.

Imagination Experiment

Rate Your Anxiety: Notice how you feel. Using a scale from 1 to 9, with 1 being very relaxed and 9 being very anxious, rate how you feel right now. Record this rating in your journal.

First Scene: Imagine sitting on the grass in a lovely little park along the edge of the woods. You are sitting on a cloth, enjoying an afternoon repast of mineral water, cheese, bread, and fruit. It is a warm spring day. Your little dog is sleeping peacefully in the thick grass next to you. You notice butterflies in nearby wildflowers. Your snack is delicious. The sun warms and soothes you as you enjoy your picnic on this lovely afternoon.

Rate Your Anxiety: Stop. Notice how you feel after imagining yourself picnicking in the park. Using the same scale as before, rate your anxiety level. Record this rating in your journal next to the first rating.

Second Scene: Imagine being at your picnic site again, enjoying a delicious lunch as you luxuriate in the warm spring sun. You notice a noise in the bushes. Your little dog looks in the direction of the noise and growls lowly. You see a large cat looking out at you from the bushes. It's a mountain lion! Petrified, you review stories you've heard about mountain lions. The cat moves a step toward you, and your little dog growls again. The lion hesitates, then turns and disappears into the woods. You sit frozen, wondering if the lion will return. Your little dog stands at alert at your side, ready to defend you.

Rate Your Anxiety: Stop. Notice how you feel after imagining the lion coming toward you. Using the same scale as before, rate your anxiety level. Record this rating in your journal next to the other ratings.

If you are like most of us, you felt calm and relaxed when imagining the lovely picnic. When you noticed the lion, your muscles probably tensed as your breathing quickened and your heart beat faster.

The preceding exercise illustrates that what you imagine can be as powerful as what is actually present at the moment. Your body responds to the images in your mind as if those images were real. What this means is that you can control your anxiety by what you imagine. And, in fact, worrywarts do just that. They make themselves anxious imagining all kinds of catastrophes—just the opposite of what they should do for themselves.

Create a Pleasant Scene

Smart worriers use imagination constructively to envision positive possibilities. By imagining something pleasant, the emotional mind thinks you are in a pleasant situation. You calm down, and anxiety dissipates as you relax.

You can lower anxiety and reduce worrying quickly by taking a few deep breaths and imagining a pleasant scene. Don't try to make up the scene on the spot when you are worrywarting; instead, have a well-developed scene ready so you know exactly what to imagine and can turn to it immediately.

A "pleasant scene" can be anything—a real situation such as sitting on the porch of your mountain cabin or an invented one like riding on a billowy white cloud. There are no limits. The only requirement is that imagining the scene soothes you. Popular pleasant scenes are walking along a beach, lying in a hammock, and walking in a meadow along a gurgling stream.

How to Script Your Scene

Select a situation that you find relaxing for your pleasant scene. Review the scene in your imagination, then write it out in your journal in one or two paragraphs.

Make It Pleasant. The most important thing about the pleasant scene is that you feel good when you imagine it. If you come across a negative, rework your scene to eliminate the negative. For example, a woman attending one of my workshops imagined picnicking in a beautiful meadow. It was very pleasant and relaxing until she realized ants were crawling on her and the food! She reworked her scene to eliminate the ants by imagining that an anteater living nearby had eaten all the ants.

Make It Detailed. Describe the setting, using as much detail as you can. The more detail you add to your scene the more real it seems to your emotional mind. Additionally, noticing a lot of detail engages your mind, keeping worrisome thoughts out.

Engage All Your Senses. The more the scene stimulates all five senses, the more powerful it will be in helping you to let the worry go for a while. Suppose your pleasant scene is walking along a secluded beach. What do you see? The sun is nearly at the zenith. Seaweed has been left when the high tide receded. Various seashells lie on the sand. There is a boat in the distance. The water is serene. A seal is swimming near the shore. What do you hear? The waves are lapping on the beach. A sea gull calls overhead. There is a tolling of a bell in the distance. What do you feel? The sun is warm on the top of your head and shoulders. You feel the rustle of your loose shirt across your skin. The sand squishes between your toes as you walk. What do you smell? The air has a salty oceany smell. You can smell the seaweed decaying. What do you taste? You run your tongue around your lips and your skin is salty. You take a drink from your water bottle and taste the cool refreshing water.

Be Active in Your Scene. Do not look at yourself as a separate character, like an actor on a movie screen. Instead, put yourself *into* the situation—imagine yourself inside your body. Imagine your scene while noticing what you see, hear, smell, and so forth, for a few minutes. Stop and add to your written description any new things you noticed when you imagined being in your pleasant scene.

Practice Going to Your Pleasant Scene

A good time to practice going to your pleasant scene is after you have relaxed by another method, such as through deep breathing or systematically relaxing your muscles. When you first awake in the morning before moving around is another good time to practice. The more you practice, the more powerful your pleasant scene will be in chasing away worry and anxiety.

Use Your Pleasant Scene to Dispel Anxiety

When you catch yourself picturing scary things, yell, "Stop!" loudly inside your head and imagine seeing a stop sign. Then purposefully switch your attention to your pleasant scene. Make it as vivid as you can. Remember to engage all your senses. When your wild mind runs back to the frightening pictures, just let them go and return to your pleasant scene.

Change Scary Pictures into Positive Possibilities

Like the wild elephant that runs out of control, worrywarts' imaginations run wildly to highly improbable pictures of extreme situations and awful disasters. The pictures are so frightening that worrywarts can work themselves into near panic attacks. They become immobilized by their scary fantasies, unable to get anything done or enjoy simple pleasures.

Imagining your pleasant scene is one way to keep out frightening pictures. Another way to deal with scary pictures is to identify and envision positive possibilities. Whereas worrywarts picture disasters and catastrophes that scare them, smart worriers use their imagination to picture positive possibilities. By doing so they soothe themselves and bring themselves back to balance.

When you catch yourself imagining catastrophic situations, get your journal and write down a description of the frightening pictures you are imagining. Use the techniques described in Chapter 11 to challenge the likelihood of such events really occurring, and write those challenges in your journal. Next, ask yourself, "What is a positive possibility in this situation?" Switch to possibility thinking and brainstorm several positive things that could happen. Write each of these in your journal.

Pick one of the possibilities that you like best and that is most likely to occur. Use the same method described above for developing a pleasant scene to flush out this possibility. Remember to add a lot of detail and engage all your senses. When you have worked up your positive fantasy of what could happen and practiced picturing it several times, you are ready to use it to drive out the frightening pictures you have been scaring yourself with. Follow the same method described above for using your pleasant scene to dispel anxiety.

As your ability grows, you can try to improvise. When you catch yourself imagining a frightening possibility, stop yourself and ask, "What is a positive possibility in this situation?" Then purposefully switch your imagination to that picture.

CHAPTER 15

You Can Worry Smarter

There is only one way to happiness and that is to cease worrying about things which are beyond the power of our will.

—EPICTETUS

Everyone worries, but some people worry smarter than others do. Smart worriers use worry to identify dangers. Then after rooting out the risks, they let go of that kind of worry and move on to soothing themselves and looking for solutions.

Smart worriers use the energy of anxiety to move them toward alternatives and solutions. You could think of it as being similar to the jujitsu master who uses the thrusting energy of an attack to throw the attacker. Similarly, smart worriers go with anxiety's energy but redirect it toward a solution, a breakthrough in thinking. Worrywarts obsess over problems, making themselves feel helpless, while smart worriers know that there is a time and place for worrying and know how to keep worry in its place with relaxation, laughter, distraction, challenges, prayer, and other ways.

Worrywarts bombard themselves with negative chatter of fuddy self-talk that fills them with fear, uncertainty, and doubt. Smart worriers stop fuddy self-talk. They talk to themselves in a friendly way, the way a supportive friend would.

Worrywarts have a one-track mind that keeps them stuck. Smart worriers are better thinkers. Smart worriers can change their thinking style to best deal with the particulars of the situation. When talking to themselves as a supportive friend would, they may use supportive thinking as they adopt a "what's working here?" type of mind-set.

Break the Worrywarting Habit

You can break free of worrywarting and become a smarter worrier. But it won't happen on its own. You must make certain changes, mostly in the way you think. The first change is to realize that you are, in fact, in control. As a worrywart you often feel helpless, but you are the only one who can get you out of worrywarting. You are responsible for making yourself happy or anxious.

Changing Is Difficult

We all know that the first step is the hardest. Of course, the second, third, and fourth steps are hard, too. But you never get to those challenges if you don't take that critical first step.

Inertia is the reason that taking the first step toward becoming a smarter worrier is so hard. Inertia is a principle of physics, which means that it is part of the physical process of the universe. The principle of inertia states that *a body at rest will tend to stay at rest, and a body in motion will tend to stay in motion.*

When you first try to make a change of any sort, you are a body at rest, at least metaphorically speaking. Inertia works against your desire to do something differently. Inertia pushes you to continue doing what you have been doing. In this case, it is easiest to continue worrywarting.

Taking the first step in a new direction is necessary to get moving toward the change you desire. That is the point of maximum resistance. Once you are in motion in a new direction—no matter how slowly—the principle of inertia can work for you because once moving you will tend to keep moving.

As an example, if your car has a dead battery, you can sometimes get it to start by pushing it with the transmission in neutral, then when it's rolling, "popping it" into second gear. When the car is at rest it takes the most effort to get the car rolling—to break the car's inertia. Once moving, it takes less effort to keep the car moving, unless you let the car stop. Then you must once again exert considerable effort to get the car moving again. On the other hand, once you get the car rolling, it takes *less effort to keep it rolling* because a body in motion tends to stay in motion.

You can break inertia by taking small steps. Changing from worrywarting to smart worrying is not all-or-nothing. Small changes add up. Remember that old saying, a journey of a thousand miles begins with the first step. Be smart. Set yourself up to succeed. Take small steps. Breathing in slowly and deeply to relax yourself is a small step that you can do any time in any place, for example. Reminding yourself to lighten up and see the humor in the situation is another small step. You might write a list of small steps you could take, if you were to take a step toward becoming a smarter worrier. Just the very act of making the list is a small step in and of itself. Then you can acknowledge yourself in a positive, supportive way for taking the step, which will help to keep the momentum you have gotten going.

Acknowledge Your Small Steps

Acknowledging yourself for taking a small step is how you keep yourself in motion. We all need pats on the back—especially in the critical first steps of change. Focus on your progress. Point out to yourself what you have done that is right. Reward yourself for trying—for taking a step. Remember that prescription: give yourself an A for effort? It's hard to change and you deserve to be recognized for making the effort—regardless of its effectiveness. List things you want. Make sure you add lots of small pleasurable things you can use as rewards for making small steps. Don't be miserly. Be generous with yourself.

Use Friendly Self-Talk

Catch fuddy-duddy talk and stop it. Talk to yourself the way a supportive friend would. Changing your self-talk is the hardest change of all. And, of course, what is worrywarting but talking to yourself in a scary way. Once again, take small steps. Ask only a small change of yourself. At first, strive simply to catch yourself worrywarting. Studying your worrywarting style is an important step. Observe what you do when you are worrywarting. Don't try to change it, just watch it. The more you know about when and how you worry, the easier it will be for you to make those small changes.

Expect Resistance

Resistance is natural. Expect it and prepare to overcome it. Resistance will work against your changing. It will stop your movement and cause you to come to rest again, so that you will have to start over with the first step. This is natural. Expect resistance and have a plan to deal with it. Expect your resolve to become a smart worrier to wane and to find yourself falling back into your old worrywarting habits. Resistance is your inertia. You overcome it by getting started, by making a beginning. Instead of worrying about finishing, focus on beginning again. Most importantly, have a plan for beginning again, and again, and again. Changing yourself takes a thousand beginnings and then more beginnings after that.

Resistance comes in many forms. The mode of resistance tends to be in your thinking. A lot of what you think—especially when worrying—is irrational, but you accept it, uncritically, as truth. You play tricks on yourself in which you pretend that you're not resisting change. Irrational, exaggerated thinking is the prose of fuddy-duddy thinking. Following are just a few ways of resisting.

Justification
A frequent resistance is justification. You make excuses for your worrywarting and why it's the only way you can respond

to the situation. Of course, there are always alternatives and options to view the situation differently. Nonetheless, you justify the way you are, which is an excuse for not changing. Brainstorming all your possibilities and keeping them in your journal can help overcome this tendency.

Procrastination

Procrastination is another resistance. You tell yourself that you will take a particular small step, but then you put off doing so. This is inertia at work. You tell yourself that you'll wait until your anxiety goes down, until you feel differently, or until someone else does something, before taking the step.

A better approach is to take a small step, one that is just enough to make a little stretch in your ability and to experience the anxiety in the process. Then when you succeed in the small step—and you make sure that you will succeed by requiring of yourself a step that you know you can achieve—the anxiety subsides. This is how you rid yourself of worrywarting and build an inner strength, which gives you the confidence to take the next step. Then each step is a little easier than the last. In the process, you create self-esteem and set yourself up to succeed.

Conflict Avoidance

Sometimes resistance is plain old avoidance. Maybe changing means you must speak up for yourself, but you want to avoid being assertive. Other times, it's making a decision—a choice—to change. Yet, doing nothing is also a decision. It's a decision to not change.

Avoidance is a marriage of inertia and fear that keeps you put—putting up with worrywarting forever. If you do the thing you are avoiding and nothing bad happens, then the fear will subside. But fear keeps you from doing it. In short, you are controlled by fear. Taking small steps—very small steps, beginning with just imagining what you would do—can help to desensitize you to fear.

Blame Others
Blaming others is an age-old way to resist changing. You tell yourself that other people are causing you to worrywart and that you can't help yourself because of things other people do. The only person you can control and can change is yourself. If you make your doing something contingent on someone else changing first, then you'll probably never change—and it will always be their fault. Instead of blaming others, always look for what *you* can do.

Overanalyzing
Getting caught up in every little detail of the worrisome situation is a subtle and insidious resistance. Analyzing risks and vulnerabilities is good—to a point. Too much analysis is not helpful; it is obsessing.

If you have a tendency to overanalyze, then you should definitely set limits. Creating a worry place, as described in Chapter 7, will help you contain this kind of runaway worry. Another powerful technique for curbing obsessing is distraction (see Chapter 19). Don't wait until you are paralyzed with worry to attempt distraction. Instead, take a small step today. Practice distraction when you are feeling good and have few worries. Then, as you gain skill and confidence, try distracting yourself from more compelling worries.

Denial

Denial is a powerful resistance. You tell yourself that worry-warting is not a problem for you—even though worrying constantly interferes with your life, a fact that you sweep aside. You are skeptical and cynical about your ability to change, so you tell yourself that it won't work anyway. Remember, it's not an all-or-nothing issue. You don't have to define yourself as a worrywart to become a smarter worrier.

That's the Way I Am

The belief that you cannot change is another resistance. Of course you can change. You can think differently; you can act differently. You can laugh; you can breathe deeply. You don't have to be trapped in worrywarting. But you must believe that you can change.

Changing is hard enough as it is. If you tell yourself that you are fixed forever, you'll have a lot of trouble getting enough motivation to make the first step. If you do this to yourself then this is the place to start: you must rewrite this self-limiting script—your self-identity as an incurable worrywart. Worrywarting is a habit, and you can change habits. Stop telling yourself and your friends that you are a worrywart. You know, *people believe what you tell them about yourself.* If you tell them that you are a worrywart, they believe you. Worse, you believe yourself! Practice describing yourself in some other way. See if you can go an entire day without saying the word *worry* to anyone.

Be Open to Change

When you catch yourself justifying, procrastinating, and blaming, recognize that you are resisting and make a plan for getting started once again toward becoming a smarter worrier. As you become more open to change, new alternatives and possibilities will emerge. Anything is possible. And among those possibilities is that you can become a smart worrier and escape the self-imposed prison of worrywarting. All it takes is one small step, a deep breath when you notice anxiety, a chuckle when you catch yourself "awfulizing," and—guess what?—you're being just a little smarter with your worry. Each little thing that you do that helps you bridle obsessive worrywarting makes you a little bit smarter. Imagine if you did one tiny thing each day, how much that would add up to in a week, a month, a year. Remember, concentrate on making a beginning and taking small steps, and each day you'll worry smart a little more and worrywart a little less. Read on for more ways to soothe yourself and to worry smarter.

PART 3

Twenty-One Ways to Soothe Yourself and Worry Smart

CHAPTER 16

Evaluate the Cost of the Worry

Stop worrying and start living.

—Dale Carnegie

Worrywarts think they can't live without worry because they believe it helps. Yet, comparing the cost of worrying to its benefits usually shows that the negative impact is greater than the value derived. You can motivate yourself to overcome worrywarting by evaluating the cost of the worry.

Is This Worry Worthwhile?

Most worrywarts don't realize the detrimental toll worrying is taking on their lives. By comparing the cost of the worry to its benefits, you can see, often for the first time, how you are operating at a loss.

The power of this exercise is amazing. You learn to step back from your worry, which helps to reduce its urgency. At the same time, you will find that in focusing your attention away from the worry onto evaluating its impact on you can be surprisingly soothing. When the costs are negative, and they usually are with worrywarting, this exercise helps you build the motivation to change.

Uncover the Fear

When you catch yourself worrywarting, don't admonish yourself to stop worrying. Instead, accept the worry and ask yourself, "What am I telling myself about this situation?" The answer to this question describes your worry—what you fear will happen relative to this situation. Record the worry on a notepad or in your journal just as you tell it to yourself.

Describe the Impact

Uncover the worry's impact on your life by asking yourself, one by one, the following questions. Take your time and record your answers below the description of your worry.

Questions

How does this worry affect my feelings?
How does this worry affect my actions?
How does this worry affect my health?
How does this worry affect my opinion of myself?
How does this worry affect my relationships?

Evaluate the Worry's Impact

Review what you have written about how the worry has affected you. Take a deep breath, step back, assume a detached frame of mind, and ask yourself, "How does this worry help or hinder me?" The answer to this question reveals the worry's cost or benefit. Take your time in coming up with answers to this important question.

CHAPTER 17

Take a Deep Breath

When I need solitude, I ... sit until my breath comes slow and gentle, and I am able to enter ... the center of my being.

—SAM KEEN, *author, professor, and philosopher*

I f you are feeling anxious and clouded by worrying, breathe deeply. Deep breathing is one of the fastest ways to quell anxiety. The key is to breathe slowly, steadily, smoothly, and deeply.

Breathing Deeply Is Relaxing

You can't be anxious and relaxed at the same time because they are what psychologists call "incompatible" responses. As with standing and sitting, you can do one or the other but not both at the same time. This means that you can effectively push anxiety out by breathing deeply.

How to Breathe Deeply

If you are breathing correctly your abdomen goes out when you breathe in, and in when you breathe out. Check that you are breathing properly by placing your hand on your abdomen, noticing it going in and out as you breathe. Stop if you feel light-headed.

Breathing Meditation

Breathe in slowly and deeply for four seconds. Then hold your breath for four seconds. Exhale slowly for four seconds. Then hold for four seconds. Repeat this sequence in a slow, even rhythm for ten minutes or until you feel calmed.

Watch your abdomen the first couple of times you breathe in and exhale out to make sure you are breathing correctly. When you have exhaled completely, try to push just a little more air out and then hold it for four seconds.

Count Inhales and Exhales

Count inhales and exhales from 1 to 4, as follows: "1 (inhale) and 2 (exhale) and 3 (inhale) and 4 (exhale)," with "and" coinciding with the hold phase. Focus all your attention on breathing and counting.

Counting inhales and exhales helps create a smooth, steady rhythm. But even more importantly, counting crowds out worrisome thoughts—because you can think only one thought at a time. Inevitably, your mind will wander back to the worry. When it does, don't scold yourself. Remember, your mind is like a wild elephant that runs away when you try to control it. When your mind wanders, just let the distracting thought go and bring your attention back to counting.

Notice How Breathing Is Soothing

Before starting, notice how you feel. What is your anxiety level? You might rate your anxiety on a scale from 1 to 9, with

1 being very low anxiety and 9 being very high anxiety, and record the rating on a notepad or in your journal.

After practicing deep breathing for ten minutes, rate your anxiety level again, using the scale from 1 to 9, and write it next to the first rating. Compare your anxiety level after the deep breathing to the level before breathing deeply for a few minutes. Do you feel more relaxed, more centered, and more in command?

Instruct Yourself

It helps to instruct yourself in a friendly way when breathing deeply to relax. You might say, "Okay, I need to relax. Just breathe in slowly. Good. Now hold it. Good." The self-instruction guides you through the exercise while crowding out worrisome thoughts.

Breathe Deeply Often

Deep breathing can be used any time and in any place. When you notice yourself feeling tense, you can relax with a few minutes of breathing and counting. Deep breathing is a powerful adjunct to other smart-worry techniques. After all, you're breathing all the time, so you may as well breathe slowly and deeply and reap the benefits.

CHAPTER 18

Relax Your Muscles

He who is of a calm and happy nature will hardly feel the pressure of age.

—PLATO, *The Republic*

Tension and worrywarting go hand in hand. Worrying makes you tense. The reverse is also true. When tense, you are inclined to worry. It is easier to relax your muscles than to relax your mind, yet when you release muscle tension you also release mental tension.

Tension Can Trigger Worrywarting

Worrywarting can make you a prisoner of the anxiety-worry cycle. The slightest twinge of anxiety can set your mind searching to uncover hidden dangers that might be causing it, and before you know it, worrywarting is in full swing. The sensation of anxiety that acts as a cue or trigger for worrying is usually tension—a tightness in the muscles. Muscle tension is an intervention point because by relaxing muscles you remove one of the catalysts for worrying.

Systematically Relax Your Muscles

Find a place where you can be comfortable and won't be disturbed for about a half hour. You might lie on your bed, on the couch, or on a futon on the floor. Sitting in an overstuffed chair is also good. Loosen your belt and any tight clothing. Kick off your shoes. You might dim the lights and play soothing music.

Begin by closing your eyes and taking a couple of slow, deep breaths. Tense and relax your muscles, one by one, starting at the top of your body and moving down to your toes. Hold the tension for about seven seconds while you study how tension feels, then release it and allow the muscle to relax. When the muscles are relaxed, try to extend the feeling of relaxation in the muscle a little further while studying how relaxation feels. Tense and relax each muscle twice before moving on to the next one.

Breathe in as you tense the muscle and breathe out as you relax. Focus your attention on the feelings of tension and relaxation. Disregard any worrisome thoughts that may intrude and return your attention to your breathing and the feelings of tension and relaxation.

Arms and Hands

■ **Hand and forearm:** Make a fist to put tension in your hand and forearm.

■ **Biceps:** Bend the arm at the elbow and make a "he-man" muscle to tense your biceps.

Face and Throat

■ **Face:** To tense your face muscles, squint your eyes, wrinkle your nose, and try to pull your whole face into a point at the center.

■ **Forehead:** Knitting or raising your eyebrows will put tension into your forehead.

■ **Cheeks:** To tense your cheeks, pull the corners of your mouth to your ears while clenching your teeth.

■ **Nose and upper lip:** With your mouth slightly open, slowly bring your upper lip down to your lower lip to tense your nose and upper lip.

■ **Mouth:** To tense your mouth, press the right corner of your mouth into your teeth and push the corner slowly toward the center of your mouth. Repeat for the left corner.

■ **Lips and tongue:** With your teeth slightly apart, press your lips together and push your tongue into the top of your mouth to put tension into your lips and tongue.

■ **Chin:** Tense your chin by crossing your arms over your chest, sticking out your chin, and turning it slowly as far as it will go to the left. Then repeat for the right side.

- **Neck:** Tense your neck by pushing your chin into your chest at the same time as pushing your head against the back of your chair (or into the bed if you are lying down) to create a counterforce.

Upper Body

- **Shoulders:** Tense the shoulders by attempting to touch your ears with your shoulders.

- **Upper back:** Push your shoulder blades together and stick out your chest to put tension in the upper back.

- **Chest:** Tense your chest by taking a deep breath and holding it in.

- **Stomach:** Pull your stomach into your spine or push it out to tense your stomach area.

Lower Body

- **Buttocks:** Buttocks are tensed by tightening them and pushing into the chair or futon.

- **Thighs:** Straighten your legs and tighten your thigh muscles to put tension into the thighs.

- **Calves:** Tense your calves by pointing your toes toward your head.

- **Toes:** Tense your toes by curling them; do this gently so they don't cramp.

Massage Your Muscle Tension Away

Slowly kneading or rubbing muscles can dissolve the tension triggered by worry. You can massage your own neck or wrist muscles or exchange a loving massage with a friend or sweetheart; or treat yourself to the luxury of a massage or body work session by a professional. As your tense muscles are soothed, so is the worried mind.

Playing relaxing music and using aromatic oil help focus your attention on the pleasing sensations of massage. Luxuriating in the warmth generated by the caring strokes helps you drift into a more relaxed state. If your mind should wander to a worrisome situation, just let it go and bring your attention back to the nurturing sensations of the massage.

Distract Yourself

This is the dog
That worried the cat
That killed the rat
That ate the malt
That lay in the house
That Jack built.

—Anonymous

There is no point in worrying about something that you can't do anything about. In fact, worrying about something that is outside your control only gets you needlessly worked up. It is smarter to distract yourself—get your mind off the worrisome situation—instead of fretting and making yourself feel helpless.

The Art of Distraction

Distraction is a technique that you've probably used intuitively all your life. Instead of trying to stop thinking about a worry, redirect your attention toward something else. Especially effective is concentrating on a lot of details. The distraction crowds the worry out. When there is less worry in your mind, you feel less anxious. It is as simple as that!

The key to the distraction technique is shifting attention toward something neutral or positive rather than trying to stop paying attention to the worry. Trying to reduce anxiety with an admonition like "I must not be anxious" rarely works. The simple process of telling yourself not to be anxious focuses attention on your anxiety, usually causing it to worsen—the opposite of what you want to accomplish.

Hypnotherapists are especially careful to phrase suggestions positively, because the unconscious mind tends to ignore negatives. A person wanting to lose weight, for example, would respond more positively to a posthypnotic suggestion that she see herself feeling good wearing a size 9, than to suggest that she not want to eat sweets.

Concentrate on Simple Mental Tasks

Even though the mind is like a high-end computer in many of its capabilities, we seem limited to concentrating on only one train of thought at a time. You can drive worry out by deliberately concentrating on something just difficult enough to take your full attention. Adding up items in your head, memorizing and repeating an excerpt from a book you like, and balancing your checkbook are examples of simple mental tasks that can drive out worry.

Count Things

Counting things drives out anxious thoughts by keeping your mind filled with counting and recounting. Find something to count, such as cracks in the wall, dots in a wallpaper design, leaves on a potted plant, or floor tiles.

Strike Up a Conversation

Some people talk to block out bothersome thoughts. We all know people who spend hours each day on the phone. If you're fearful about flying, for example, you can distract yourself by talking with the person in the next seat. Social conversation has the greatest effect on worrying when you are speaking rather than listening. The best topics are those that make you feel good, which may include stories of past triumphs or recollections of good times. In general, it's best to avoid topics related to anxiety-provoking situations.

CHAPTER 20

Take a Walk

Little by little one walks far.
—Peruvian proverb

When feeling anxious, taking a walk can make you feel better. When you are more relaxed and level-headed, you can revisit the worrisome situation to look for a solution and develop a plan of action for dealing with it. This is the approach smart worriers take.

Walking Stimulates Endorphins

Taking a walk reduces the anxiety accompanying worry by increasing endorphin levels. Endorphins are brain hormones that reduce pain and anxiety. Similar in chemical structure to opiates, endorphins induce a state of comfort and well-being. Physical exercise stimulates your brain to produce endorphins.

Exercise is not the only stimulant for the production of endorphins. Being in the presence of one's beloved prompts their production. Dogs and cats have higher levels of endorphins, for example, after being petted and playing with their owners.

Like real opiates, you can develop an addiction to endorphins and suffer withdrawal symptoms when deprived of them. When you are away from a loved one, you suffer, in part, because of the reduction in endorphin levels. Similarly, pets that normally receive a lot of affection from their owners will exhibit withdrawal symptoms when separated from them. Withdrawal symptoms include anxiety and depression, and the endorphins produced when taking a walk can serve as an antidote.

Walking Off Your Worry

Move briskly while swinging your arms to the rhythm of your pace. Exercising your muscles releases built-up tension. Breathing relaxes you. Breathe in and out deeply in sync with your movement. Worriers walk with their shoulders hunched, which constricts breathing, and their heads lowered, keeping their attention focused inward. Holding your head up and your shoulders back makes you breathe more deeply. Look outward. Engage your senses. Notice what you see. Listen to the sounds around you. Smell odors. Feel the texture of your clothes brushing your body and the ground under your feet. Walk long enough to unwind.

Focus your mind on the activity of walking and observing your surroundings. When a worrisome thought intrudes, passively disregard it and return your attention to walking and watching.

CHAPTER 21

Smile and Laugh

*Pack up your troubles in your old kit-bag and
smile, smile, smile.*

—George Asat

When you are tense and pent up with worry, smile. Smiling and laughing release vast amounts of stored emotions, enabling you to regain balance and defuse the worry.

Practice Smiling and Laughing

When you smile you send a message to your emotional brain that there must be something funny happening. It primes the pump, so to speak. Remember the old saying, "Smile and the whole world smiles with you." When you smile you raise your spirits and those of people around you. When you smile you worry less. Things don't seem as catastrophic. To a certain degree, you can generate positive feelings simply by smiling.

Laughing functions in a similar way, providing relief from tension. We've all been in a tense situation where someone made a joke or burst out laughing and the tension was released, making it easier for everyone to get on with the task at hand. Just the mere act of laughing releases tension and chases away worries. You can be tense or you can be relaxed, but you can't be tense and relaxed simultaneously because the two conditions are incompatible.

Here are two fun ways to chase worries away with smiles and laughter, inspired by C. W. Metcalf, author of *Lighten Up: Survival Skills for People Under Pressure*.

The Smile Exercise

Assume a comfortable sitting position. Count to three and on "three," stand up and smile the biggest smile that you can. Make sure to take a deep breath and to smile so big that your teeth show. Sit back down and repeat the exercise several times. The fun of this exercise can be increased by doing it regularly with your family at home or with co-workers at the office. When you feel worrywarting coming on, take a deep breath, stand up, and smile broadly several times.

Carry Foolish Photos

Assemble a collection of photographs of you looking and acting ridiculous. An easy, quick way to do this is in one of those photo booths you find in five-and-dime stores and on oceanside boardwalks. Make four snapshots of yourself looking silly. Stick out your tongue; squint your eyes; bare your teeth like a vicious dog. Make the most ridiculous faces you can conjure up. Keep your foolish photos on your cell phone or in your purse or wallet to use as a tool to regain a sense of humor. Whenever you catch yourself worrying about what others might think or how foolish you may have acted, take out your foolish photos and look at them to remember to laugh.

CHAPTER 22

Say a Little Prayer

Yea, though I walk in the valley of the shadow of death, I shall fear no evil.

—PSALMS 23

W hen you feel helpless before a worry, say a little prayer. Focusing your attention on the prayer while disregarding intruding thoughts elicits the relaxation response, which brings you back to balance physically, mentally, and spiritually. Saying a prayer is soothing.

Praying Builds Hope

The power of prayer is often scoffed at in the modern world. Yet, according to a 1990 Gallup poll, 95 percent of Americans believe in God, and 76 percent of Americans pray regularly. Believing in something immortal and enduring is deeply soothing to both psyche and body. Faith that there is a larger meaning, a grander scheme, builds hope. A sense that things will turn out for the good counters worry and soothes the soul.

Say a Prayer

Saying a prayer repetitively is a powerful way to drive out worries. Your mind can focus on only one thing at a time, so repeating your prayer crowds the worry out. You might recite a traditional prayer, such as The Lord's Prayer, or a psalm, such as The Lord Is My Shepherd, or a prayer you've written. You might repeat a poem or a meaningful word, like "love." Keep your mind on the words of the prayer as you repeat it over and over. When a worry intrudes, passively disregard it as you return your attention to saying your prayer.

Join a Prayer Group

The feelings of connectedness and hope you gain from praying with others makes your prayers more effective in soothing your worries and bringing you back to balance. There are two kinds of prayer groups: one where members gather together to pray, and another where members agree to pray separately but at the same time for the same purpose, such as healing a sick friend.

Expect Miracles

When worrying about what awful things could happen, say to yourself, "Stop! I will expect a miracle." Then deliberately imagine a miraculous occurrence in the worrisome situation. Make a prayer of the miracle and create a mental picture of the good it brings. When you catch your mind running back to the scary images, stop yourself again, say, "I will expect a miracle," and repeat your prayer while picturing good things that could happen.

CHAPTER 23

Find the Joy

Don't hurry, don't worry. You're only here for a short visit.
So be sure to stop and smell the flowers.

—WALTER HAGEN, *championship golfer*

If worry is making life look gray, look for the joy. There is always a joy—the whistle of a bird, the smell of salt in the sea breeze. Noticing the joy in the moment lightens your worry load.

The Discipline of Joy

Finding joy in living will not happen spontaneously. You must discipline your mind to look for it. Humor expert C. W. Metcalf says a disciplined joy in living is a *skill* that allows those who possess it to draw strength from circumstances that would defeat other people. You must train your wild mind to find joy in living, regardless of worrisome situations.

You can choose to feel joyful or you can choose to sit around worrying. Just because worrying feels natural, it doesn't mean that it is natural to give your free time over to worry. It may seem automatic and natural, while doing joyful things feels forced and artificial. But that is because worrying is a well-worn bad habit. With discipline and practice, being joyful, even in the face of difficulties, can feel natural, too.

Look for the Joy

Joy is an emotion of delight. When you catch yourself in a worry, stop and remind yourself, in a friendly way, to look for the joy in the moment. What beauty do you see? What feels good? What is satisfying? If you find this difficult, and most worrywarts do, then you need to train your wild mind to have a disciplined joy in living. A joy list can help.

Create a Joy List

A joy list is just that—a list of joyful activities and situations. It is a great tool for helping rediscover your joy. Start a list of joys in your journal. Note on this list anything that makes you smile, laugh, or feel good. Especially important are the small things, the brief moments of joy. The refreshing feeling of a breeze on your cheek on a hot summer day, the aroma of your favorite pot roast cooking for dinner, the silky sensuous feeling of your cat's fur as you pet it—the possibilities are endless. Enjoy!

CHAPTER 24

Avoid Drinking Coffee

All the things I really like to do are either immoral,
illegal, or fattening.

—ALEXANDER WOOLLCOTT

S ome worrywarts drink six to twelve or more cups of coffee a day. However, the stimulation from caffeine can increase your anxiety, making you worry more, and even pushing you to the brink of a panic attack. When worried, avoid drinking coffee—as well as other beverages high in caffeine, such as colas.

Caffeine Is a Stimulant

The caffeine in coffee is a powerful stimulant. In one study, for example, experienced cocaine users couldn't tell powdered caffeine from cocaine. You can overdose on caffeine. Yes, caffeine is a drug. After only five to six cups, sensitive people can experience caffeine intoxication, which includes such symptoms as nervousness, excitement, restlessness, heart palpitations, insomnia, and rambling thought and speech. In fact, the symptoms of "caffeinism" are essentially indistinguishable from those of anxiety neurosis. People drinking eight to fourteen cups of coffee daily score high on anxiety tests and report dizziness, apprehension, butterflies in the stomach, restlessness, frequent episodes of diarrhea, and sleep problems. Doctors' reports indicate that as many as 25 percent of patients with anxiety disorders dramatically recovered after doing nothing more than giving up caffeine and cigarettes, which contain nicotine, another powerful stimulant.

Test the Impact of Coffee

If you think caffeine might be contributing to your worrying, you can do a test. Take a few moments to notice yourself and how you feel right now. Using a scale from 1 to 9, with 9 being very anxious, rate your anxiety level. Keep this rating in your journal as a comparison point or "baseline." Count the number of cups of coffee you typically drink and cut back by 50 percent for a few days. Once or twice a day, rate your anxiety on the same scale. Record these scores next to your initial anxiety ratings. After several days, review your anxiety data. Did your anxiety rating go down? If it did, you can probably benefit from a permanent cutback in drinking coffee.

Avoid Caffeine

Drink caffeine-free tea with honey, sweetened warm milk, and other soothing beverages to counter the anxiety caused by your worry. Caffeine is widely used in soft drinks and over-the-counter medicines, so read the labels to check for caffeine. Also, be careful about eating chocolate because it contains substantial amounts of caffeine and another stimulant, theobromine.

CHAPTER 25

Change Shoulds to Preferences

> *Success is getting what you want. Happiness is wanting what you get.*
>
> —Anonymous

Worrywarts worry about what they "should" do, what others "ought" to do, and what "must" happen. Shoulds, oughts, and musts are epidemic among worrywarts. While it may seem silly when reading it here, enormous numbers of people make themselves sick worrying about what they "should" do and berate themselves and other people when something does not happen as it "should." You can lessen the grip of a worry by discovering your hidden shoulds and changing them to preferences.

Shoulds Are Imperatives

Shoulds become tyrants because they are demands—must-dos. When something doesn't go as it "should," worrywarts view it as awful and tell themselves that they can't stand it. They are caught in a cycle of perfectionism, striving for unrealistic standards. They entangle themselves in judgmental self-talk about what they and others "should" be doing—which is often at odds with their own best interest.

When a should is not met, we tend to view the situation as awful, terrible, and bad, which triggers anxiety and worrywarting, whereas when a preference is not forthcoming it is a disappointment, but not a disaster.

Catch and Replace Shoulds

You can reduce your worries by uncovering shoulds, oughts, and musts in your worry. Start by making a "should list" in your journal. On the left side of the page, list criteria you expect yourself and others to meet that are implicit in your worry. For example, if your son is late returning home with the family car, the hidden *should* may be, "He *should* call me if he's late. He didn't call and that is awful!" Then convert each *should* into a preference and write it next to the *should* it replaces. For the example of the son being late, the preference statement would be, "I *prefer* that he call me when he's late. He didn't call and I don't like it." Look at the following examples:

Should	*Preference*
I should always look good.	I like to look good.
John should make more money.	I prefer that John made more money.
I should exercise more.	I would like to exercise more.
Alice should keep the house cleaner.	I prefer that Alice keep the house cleaner.
Everyone should like me.	I prefer that everyone like me.

Stop "Shoulding" Yourself

Thinking in shoulds is just a bad thinking habit, one that is fairly easy to change by substituting the word *prefer* for *should*. Substituting preferences for shoulds is a small change that has a big impact because it changes your self-talk. It shifts the focus from imperatives to preferences; from worrywarting demands to new and hopeful possibilities.

CHAPTER 26

Count Worry Beads

Don't worry, be happy.

—MEHER BABA

Rosaries have been used for thousands of years as an adjunct to praying. Counting beads, as you hold them one by one, engages your fingers and your mind. When you're fidgety and tense, or bothered by intrusive thoughts, count worry beads.

What Are Worry Beads?

Worry beads are a string of twenty or so bean-sized beads on a leather or velvet string, with the ends tied together creating a circle of beads, with a knot where the ends meet. The object is to keep your fingers busy while you fill your mind with words that crowd out the worry.

How to Worry Your Beads

Keep your worry beads in your pocket or purse. When a worry threatens to take over your mind, let the beads do the worrying! Here's how it works. While holding the first bead, next to the knot on your string of beads, between your forefinger and thumb, say, "One," silently to yourself. Then, while holding the second bead between your fingers, say, "Two," silently to yourself. Proceed in this fashion through all the beads on the string, holding the bead between your fingers and counting silently to yourself. When you reach the knot, you can begin counting the beads over again. As alternatives, instead of counting, you can say a short prayer or a meaningful affirmation—such as Meher Baba's famous mantra, "Don't worry, be happy"—silently to yourself, repeating it as you hold each bead individually.

Mantras and Chants

Instead of counting, you can use a mantra. A mantra is a sound or phrase that you repeat silently to yourself. Sometimes the mantra has a special meaning, such as "God is beautiful. God is good." Other times, as in the practice of transcendental meditation, or TM, it is a specific sound, like a vowel, that the teacher tells you to repeat silently. Chants are mantras said out loud, repetitively.

The purpose of the mantra or chant is to drive out other thoughts. This works because you can think in words about only one thing at a time. When concentrating on saying the mantra or the chant repetitively, worrisome thoughts are blocked out.

CHAPTER 27

Eat a Sweet

Sugar in the gourd and honey in the horn, I never was so happy since the hour I was born.

—From the song "Turkey in the Straw"

People give friends and loved ones candies because eating sweets feels good. Not only does candy taste wonderful, but eating sweets has a soothing biochemical effect on the brain. You can calm anxiety by eating food rich in starch and sugar.

Eating Sweets Makes You Feel Good

Sugar plays a pivotal role in the brain's manufacturing of serotonin, often called the "feel good" neurotransmitter. Neurotransmitters are chemicals that carry messages from one nerve cell to another. Serotonin works to calm operations of the brain. When its levels are adequate, you feel pleasantly relaxed and safe, whereas low levels of serotonin are associated with depression, irritability, and trouble sleeping.

Kids, who are usually cheerful, have plenty of serotonin. As you grow older, however, your serotonin can run low due to diet and general aging. Old folks tend to be much grouchier than little kids, and low levels of serotonin are part of the reason. You don't have to be older to experience low serotonin. It can also be depleted by dieting and eating poorly.

Increasing serotonin levels has a tranquilizing effect similar to that experienced when taking the popular antidepressant Prozac. Prozac works by inhibiting a process called reuptake, or the removal of used serotonin from the brain, so that levels remain high.

Serotonin enhances feelings of security, courage, assertiveness, self-worth, calm, flexibility, resilience—all of which have the effect of making one feel safe—a feeling worrywarts long for but rarely get to enjoy for long. You don't have to take Prozac, however, to enjoy the effects of serotonin because your brain manufactures it out of nutrients found in common foods. The problem is that certain nutrients needed to manufacture serotonin must cross the barrier into the brain. Sugar facilitates the transfer process.

Calm Yourself by Eating Sugar or Carbs

Eating sugar and carbohydrates, which are converted into sugar, has a tranquilizing effect. When you want to calm down, eat carbohydrates including potatoes, pasta, bread, beans, and cereal.

For the fastest tranquilizing effect, drink a beverage high in honey or sugar. A sugary drink will calm you in about five minutes. Sucking on pure sugar candy like gumdrops, caramels, mints, or lollipops is also fast acting. Other calming drinks include caffeine-free teas, such as chamomile or peppermint, with generous amounts of honey or sugar.

Sebastian remembered an experience from his childhood where sugar saved the day. "When I was a boy in Brazil my sister, Gabby, was bitten by a chimp in the zoo. Mama acted fast to pull Gabby away from the chimp and took her straight to the hospital for stitches and shots. By that time, Mama was a nervous wreck, hyperventilating, as she paced and mumbled. A kind nurse gave Mama 'medicine' to make her feel better—a glass of sugar-water—which she insisted that Mama drink completely. Within a couple of minutes, Mama was her old calm self."

Eating carbohydrate-rich bread takes about forty-five minutes to slow you down. Don't mix protein with the carbohydrates, such as putting milk on cereal or cheese on the bread, because the protein will counteract the carbohydrate's calming effect. Low-fat carbohydrates are better than those that are high in fat, which take longer to work. Avoid chocolate, which is high in fat and contains caffeine.

As a note of caution, this technique for soothing yourself should be used in moderation. Don't "pork out," as too many carbs may not be healthy. Remember, this is one of many techniques to experiment with to see what helps soothe your worries.

CHAPTER 28

Take a Warm Bath

*I have had more uplifting thoughts soaking in
comfortable baths than I have ever had in any
cathedral.*

—EDMUND WILSON

There is something especially soothing about being in
warm water; perhaps it's a memory of the security of
being in the womb. As heat from the water penetrates
into your muscles, tension melts, anxiety recedes, and worries
float away. When you are feeling overwhelmed with worry, try
taking a warm bath.

Prepare for Your Bath

Check the stove, lock the doors, set the alarm, turn off the
ringer on your phone, and do anything else you would do
before going to bed. Warm up your bathroom. Think of what
you'll wear after your bath, and hang it in your bathroom. Put
towels next to the bath. Lay out a bath mat.

Use Warm Water

Find the temperature you prefer. For most people it is between 99
and 102 degrees. Test the water temperature several times as you

fill the bath. Remember that your hand can take more heat than the rest of your body, so be careful that the water is not too hot.

Perfume Your Bath

Add scented oils to your bath to create an atmosphere of serenity. Their essence combines with the steam rising from the hot water to fill the bathroom with pleasing aromas. Smells stimulate the emotions through the limbic system, the most ancient part of the brain, which is why they have such a powerful effect on the emotions.

Lavender is the traditional bath oil because it has a calming effect that relieves anxiety. Its antispasmodic properties work directly on the muscles to release tension.

Worry-Soothing Bath Oil Blend
4 drops chamomile oil
4 drops lavender oil
2 drops orange oil
1 drop tea tree oil

Dim the Light

Just as a stage production uses light to set the mood for the play, you can create a serene atmosphere with soft dim light in your bathroom. Low yellow light is especially soothing, as it relaxes the mind. Candles are good because they make a flickering light that has a hypnotic effect.

Play Comforting Music

Listening to low soft music enhances the mood of serenity. An instrumental with a simple, repetitive melody and a slow, even beat is a good choice.

Focus on the Good Feeling

As you settle into your bath, focus your attention on the soothing feeling of the warm water. In your thoughts talk to yourself the way a supportive friend would to comfort you, encouraging you to relax and enjoy your bath. If the worry intrudes, dismiss it with passive disregard and switch your attention back to the good feeling of the warm water on your skin.

Visualize a Pleasant Scene

Picture in your mind a pleasant scene, one that is comforting and relaxing. If you imagine floating on a cloud or in water, for example, the flowing motion of the bath will make the scene more real in your imagination.

CHAPTER 29

Imagine a Happy Ending

[O]ur life is what our thoughts make it.

—MARCUS AURELIUS

A happy ending is far more likely than the scary things worrywarts imagine. The possibility of a happy ending gives hope, which keeps worry from running wild. When you are worried something bad will happen, stop and imagine a happy ending.

Imagining a Happy Ending Gives Hope

When you sit around worrying and imagining unlikely disastrous happenings, you make yourself sick with worry for no good reason. The fact is that most situations turn out okay in the end. So why not imagine a happy ending? Your emotional brain responds to what you imagine as if it were real. When you imagine disasters, you feel frightened and helpless; whereas imagining a happy ending builds hope and an expectation that all will be well in the end. Worry feeds on fear, while hope keeps worry in its place. There is always hope, and it is smarter to hope for the best than to expect the worst.

Script a Happy Ending

When you catch yourself imagining awful happenings in a situation, stop and ask yourself, "What would be a happy ending to this situation?" Like a novelist, write out the happy ending on paper or in your journal. Then play out the happy ending in your mind and watch what happens. Strive to actually see the positive event happening. As ideas come to you, add more detail to the scenario. Think in terms of your five senses. What will you see during the happy ending? What will you hear? Feel? Smell? Taste? Whenever the worrisome situation comes to mind, take a deep slow breath and deliberately imagine the happy ending you have written.

CHAPTER 30

Do a Good Deed

The time to be happy is now. The place to be happy is here. The way to be happy is to make others so.

—ROBERT INGERSOLL

People who do good deeds experience a "helper's high." When helping someone in need, you gain a sense of meaning that makes you feel better about yourself. When worried, you can soothe yourself by remembering your helpful acts, which brings back the feeling of well-being you had at the time you were helping.

Helping Others Helps You

Whether fretting over personal inadequacies or bad things happening, worrywarts get stuck in their anxieties. When you help someone, your focus of concern shifts away from yourself and toward another person.

The very act of helping someone can channel the anxious energy driving the worrying into benefiting someone in need. In the process of helping, you get a sense of meaning and empowerment that builds confidence and puts worries in their place. The good feelings that ensue soothe you and give a sense of being more centered.

Be Helpful

Create meaning in your life by helping others. Opportunities to help people are all around you. Do a good deed. Visit a lonely senior. Help a child with homework. Run an errand for a friend. Volunteer for a church group.

Practice Acts of Kindness

Help yourself and others to feel better and be happier by practicing acts of kindness. Keep an eye out for opportunities to do something kind. Smile at a stranger. Give your seat on the bus to someone. Leave a flower on the desk of a co-worker. Send a cheerful e-mail to a relative. Pay a stranger's order at a lunch counter. The possibilities are infinite!

Keep a Good Deeds Journal

After you've done something helpful or kind, write a description of it in your journal. Include how it benefited the person you helped and how that person felt about it. Pay particular attention to describing how you felt when you were being helpful.

Relive Your Good Deeds

When you begin to worry and feel despairing, relive your good deeds. Reread accounts of your helpfulness, then close your eyes and, in your imagination, relive the time when you were helping someone. See yourself being kind and watch how it helped. Remember how you felt when you were helpful, and enjoy the sense of meaningfulness you experience.

CHAPTER 31

Joke About the Worry

Situation Normal: All Fouled Up (SNAFU).
—World War II army saying

The popular 1970s TV series "M*A*S*H" demonstrates the power of humor to keep people sane and effective under the extreme pressures of wartime. Finding humor in a crisis takes looking at it in a different way and appreciating the absurd. Joke about the worrisome situation to gain a new perspective and feel better.

Joking Releases Anxiety

Finding a creative solution to a worrisome problem takes playing with ideas, but when you worrywart, your mind freezes up and you fixate on your fears. Like a dog with its eyes riveted on a scrap of meat on its master's plate, your mental eye similarly fixes on the fear, unable to look at other ideas. Poking fun at the worrisome situation is like a shock that confuses the fixed mind, forcing it to look elsewhere. Once freed from fixation, you might see creative alternatives.

Devise a Comic Routine

Some of the best comedians learned to use humor as a means of coping with problems in their lives, making their embarrassments, worries, and failures into jokes. Seeing the absurdity in worry takes looking from a fresh perspective—breaking out of your thinking rut. Once you've seen the worry as absurd, you've broken its grip on you. When you stop worrywarting and awfulizing with all of their extreme negativity—even briefly—you give yourself a few moments of relief from the worry and its accompanying anxiety.

Step back from your worry to consider how you might turn the situation into a comic routine. Ask yourself, what's funny here? Think of amusing ways to describe your worry to someone else. What is absurd about the situation? Exaggerate something that is mildly funny so that it becomes ridiculous. Of course, worrywarting itself is absurd, so you can always satirize the worrywarting, if not the actual worry. After you have created your comic routine, find someone—your spouse, a friend, a co-worker—to try it out on.

Give your audience permission to laugh at your absurd worrywart routine. Make sure you also laugh. You'll find the heartier you laugh, the lighter the worry becomes.

CHAPTER 32

Rock Yourself

Rock your stress away.

—ROCKING CHAIR MANUFACTURER SLOGAN

W hen an infant cries, most people instinctively want to rock it. Even though you may think of rocking as being good only for little babies, it also has a powerful calming effect on adults. When you feel shaken up by worry, rocking yourself can soothe you, allowing the worry to drift away.

Being Rocked Is Soothing

Engaging in a repetitive activity has a lulling, sometimes even a numbing effect. If you recall the movie *Rainman*, the autistic man played by Dustin Hoffman often engaged in repetitive, rocking activities, such as stepping back and forth from one foot to the other in a robotlike fashion as he said meaningless phrases over and over. While there is a lot of controversy surrounding autism, psychologists generally believe that the rocking and other repetitive behaviors serve to soothe the autistic person's extreme anxiety.

Repetitive activity is an effective relaxant for all people. Focusing your attention on a repetitive activity while passively disregarding intruding thoughts is the essential condition for eliciting the relaxation response (see Chapter 13). Once you relax and get out of your head and into your body, you will soon find it easier to disregard the worrisome thoughts fluttering around your mind.

Rock Yourself

Even though you are grown up and your mom is no longer around to rock you to sleep, you can always rock yourself for comfort. Rocking can take many forms, but basically it is any repetitive back-and-forth motion. Rocking in a favorite rocking chair is a common self-rocking technique. Another enjoyable way to rock yourself is swaying back and forth to music that has a quick, even beat. Or you can do a simple exercise such as jumping jacks, stepping up and down on a stair, or jogging. If you are more sedentary, knitting or crocheting might be a good choice. These "meditations-in-motion" soothe anxiety while lulling your mind into letting go of the worry. The worry will sneak back in, especially at first. When it does, disregard it and bring your attention back to the rocking.

CHAPTER 33

Count Your Blessings

Keep your face to the sunshine and you cannot see the shadow.

—HELEN KELLER

You always have reasons to be thankful. When your worries seem so great that you feel everything is lost, it helps to count your blessings.

Look on the Bright Side

No one's life is free of problems; even the most blessed and saintly person has worries. It is your power of attention that makes them great or small. By shining the light of your attention on a worrisome situation, you see only the worry, while the good things in your life lie forgotten in the dark. It doesn't have to be this way. Even though you have problems, you are not required to live a bleak life of worry and suffering. By shining the light of your attention on the good things in your life, you can feel better.

It is easy to forget that you choose where to focus your attention. When you look at the good things in your life, positive feelings will fill up your attention.

List Good Things You Have

On a sheet of paper write the heading "My Blessings" and below it list all the good things you have despite the worry of the moment. Make sure to add the small things that make you happy that you may be taking for granted. Don't forget your health, which is, of course, central to your well-being. List your friends and remember your pets, if you have any. Also include your talents, especially those things you do almost naturally.

Imagine a Life Without Blessings

Suppose all of the good things that bring you happiness have been taken away from you. Imagine what life would be like without them. Allow yourself to feel the emptiness for several moments.

Recognize Your Good Fortune

Imagine getting back one good thing on your list of blessings. Notice how having this blessing enriches your life. Say a prayer of gratitude as you feel a sense of appreciation for this blessing. Imagine getting back a second good thing in your life, your second blessing. Again, immerse yourself in feeling grateful. In this manner, count your blessings one by one and appreciate each of them.

CHAPTER 34

Make a List

> *Confront your fears, list them, get to know them,*
> *and only then will you be able to put them aside*
> *and move ahead.*

> —JERRY GILLIES, *Creative Affirmations*

W hen you are overwhelmed with worry and you
don't know what to do or where to start, make a
list. With a list you can make order out of a con-
fusing situation. Breaking a problem into specific items makes
it more manageable. You get a handle on it, gaining a sense of
control.

Making a List Gives You a Handle on Things

The power of "to-do" lists for helping to think things through,
identify steps, make decisions, and get started is tremendous.
When you are overwhelmed by the magnitude of a worrisome
situation, a list can help tame it. Listing concerns driving a
worry, for example, can get them out of your head and onto
paper so that you don't have to dwell on them any longer. On
paper they become focused and concrete. You can do something about each item on the list if you want to. Even when
nothing is resolved, lists help focus problems and make them
finite. The mere act of writing concerns down creates a safety
zone between you and your thoughts, so that you don't feel so
possessed by them.

How to Work on Worries with a List

Select a particular aspect of the worry or the worrisome situation that you want to tackle. When you feel overwhelmed with anxiety, it can be a soothing release to simply list all of the possible causes, for example. It might be helpful in thinking the worry through to list all the events that have happened leading up to the present. Your list can be a series of names, words, phrases, or incomplete sentences relative to a particular category you are enumerating.

Be creative with your list making. You can list assumptions underlying your concerns, for example. Experiment with listing expectations, wishes, joys, things that make you happy, desires, goals, successes, and secrets. Sometimes it is helpful to list the positives of something in one column and the negatives in a second column. When completed, a comparison of the two can be quite revealing. Other dichotomy-type lists might include successes and failures, hopes and fears, what makes you happy or unhappy, your priorities as compared to someone else's priorities.

Go ahead and experiment. After you have written down your worrisome thoughts, you can rate them, organize them, or delete them. All these actions are empowering because they put you back in control.

Practice Underreacting

What, me worry?

—Alfred E. Neuman, *Mad Magazine*

Worrisome self-talk generates anxiety and gets in the way of finding solutions. Helpful self-talk, the way a supportive friend would talk to you, is more balanced and usually downplays the risks in the situation. Lucinda Bassett, author of *From Panic to Power*, refers to this downplaying self-talk as "underreactive statements" as compared to the fuddy self-talk that triggers overreacting. Following are examples of underreactive statements.

Underreactive Statements

This is no big deal.

This will pass.

It's just anxiety. It will go away.

Don't sweat the small stuff.

Ten years from now I won't remember this.

It just doesn't matter.

This isn't an emergency.

It's not my problem.

This is not worth getting upset over.

It's only money. It's not my arm.

So what?

When you hear yourself saying, "Oh, no! What will I do?" or "Oh, my gawd, this is awful!" your emotional brain believes you are facing a real crisis and overreacts. Actually, it's easier to function in difficult situations, even emergencies, when you are calmer than when you are panicking. When you talk to yourself in a friendly way using underreactive statements, you react less. Your thinking is clearer so that you can focus on the problem at hand and think it through more easily. While fuddy self-talk tends to use overreactive statements, friendly self-talk uses underreactive statements like the ones in the list above.

When you catch yourself getting worked up, stop and ask yourself, "How can I underreact? What can I say to downplay this situation?" Remember to ask yourself the question in the same way a friend would ask it.

CHAPTER 36

Watch a Funny Movie

From the moment I picked your book up until the moment I put it down, I could not stop laughing. Someday I hope to read it.

—GROUCHO MARX

When you are stuck in a worry, watching a funny movie can help lighten up your mood. The comedy changes your frame of mind, while your laughter dispels anxiety. When you feel depressed by a worrisome situation and unable to find a creative approach for handling it, watch a funny movie.

Watching a Funny Movie Opens Your Mind

Researchers from Cornell University showed that after seeing a funny movie, people demonstrated more creative flexibility, whereas people who did not see the comedy suffered from "functional fixedness" on problem assignments. When worrying, you get stuck in a mental rut, unable to break out of your fixed viewpoint. Comedy is created with dissonance, contradictions, and contrasts, all of which help to open your mind.

Watching a Funny Movie Is Good Medicine

Norman Cousins, the famous motivational speaker, attributed his remarkable recovery from a particularly painful form of cancer to massive doses of humor, which generated positive emotions. He made the discovery that ten minutes of genuine belly laughter had an anesthetic effect that enabled him to get a couple of hours of pain-free sleep. Based on Cousins's findings, several metropolitan hospitals introduced laugh programs with funny movies as an adjunct to conventional therapy.

Watch Funny Movies and Laugh

The classic movies of Groucho Marx, Charlie Chaplin, Abbott and Costello, and Bob Hope are good choices. Don't just smile at the funny scenes. Laugh out loud. Laughing generates endorphins, a brain hormone that promotes good feelings. Avoid suspenseful movies and those with violence, which will stimulate anxiety and set you to worrying again.

Build a Cartoon Library

If there's a particular worry that plagues you, such as fear of flying or paying your bills, for example, collect cartoons and jokes lampooning the subject. *Reader's Digest* has a wealth of jokes and is a good place to look. *The New Yorker* magazine is known for its numerous poignant cartoons. When you feel a worry about flying or bill paying coming on, get out your humor collection and entertain yourself by reading over your favorite jokes and cartoons.

Babior, Shirley, and Carol Goldman. *Overcoming Panic Attacks: New Strategies to Free Yourself from Worry and Fear.* Duluth, MN: Pfeifer-Hamilton, 1996.

Bassett, Lucinda. *From Panic to Power: Proven Techniques to Calm Your Anxiety, Conquer Your Fears, and Put You in Control of Your Life.* New York: HarperCollins, 1997.

Bassett, Lucinda. *Life Without Limits.* New York: HarperCollins, 2001.

Benson, Herbert. *Timeless Healing: The Power and Biology of Belief.* New York: Scribner, 1996.

Bourne, Edmund J. *The Anxiety and Phobia Workbook.* Oakland, CA: New Harbinger, 1990.

Burns, David D. *Feeling Good: The New Mood Therapy.* New York: Avon, 1980.

Burns, David D. *Ten Days to Self-Esteem.* New York: William Morrow, 1993.

Butler, Gillian, and Tony Hope. *Managing Your Mind: The Mental Fitness Guide.* Oxford, UK: Oxford University Press, 1995.

Butler, Pamela E. *Talking to Yourself: Learning the Language of Self-Support.* New York: Harper & Row, 1981.

Carnegie, Dale. *How to Stop Worrying and Start Living.* New York: Vermilion, 1990.

Carper, Jean. *Food: Your Miracle Medicine: How Food Can Prevent and Cure over 100 Symptoms and Problems.* New York: HarperCollins, 1993.

Cousins, Norman. *Head First: The Biology of Hope.* New York: Dutton, 1989.

de Ropp, Robert S. *The Master Game.* New York: Delacorte Press, 1968.

Fry, William F., Jr., and Waleed a Salameh, eds. *Handbook of Humor and Psychotherapy: Advances in the Clinical Use of Humor.* Sarasota, FL: Professional Resource Press, 1987.

Goleman, Daniel. *Emotional Intelligence: Why It Can Matter More than IQ.* New York: Bantam Books, 1995.

Hallowell, Edward M. *Worry: Hope and Help for a Common Condition.* New York: Ballantine, 1998.

Hazlett-Stevens, Holly. *Women Who Worry Too Much: How to Stop Worry and Anxiety from Ruining Relationships, Work and Fun.* Oakland, CA: New Harbinger, 2005.

Hutchison, Michael. "Listening to the Brain: Mind Tech and the Remaking of the Self." *The Journal of Mind Technology,* Vol. 2, No. 4 (Dec 1994): 4–9.

Jampolsky, Gerald G. *Love Is Letting Go of Fear.* New York: Bantam, 1981.

Keyes, Ken, Jr. *Taming Your Mind.* St. Mary, KY: Living Love Publications, 1975.

Kramer, Peter D., *Listening to Prozac: A Psychiatrist Explores Antidepressant Drugs and the Remaking of the Self.* New York: Penguin, 1994.

Leahy, Robert L. *The Worry Cure: Seven Steps to Stop Worry from Stopping You.* New York: Three Rivers, 2006.

Lejeune, Chad. *The Worry Trap: How to Free Yourself from Worry and Anxiety Using Acceptance and Communication Therapy.* Oakland, CA: New Harbinger, 2007.

Luks, Allan. *The Healing Power of Doing Good: The Health and Spiritual Benefits of Helping Others.* New York: Fawcett Columbine, 1992.

Martorano, Joseph T., and John P. Kildahl. *Beyond Negative Thinking: Reclaiming Your Life Through Optimism.* New York: Avon, 1989.

McGinnis, Alan Loy. *The Power of Optimism.* New York: HarperCollins, 1993.

Mehrabian, Albert. *Public Places, Private Spaces: The Psychology of Work, Play and Living Environments.* New York: Basic Books, 1976.

Metcalf, C. W., and Roma Felible. *Lighten Up: Survival Skills for People Under Pressure.* Boston: Addison-Wesley, 1992.

Midwest Center for Stress and Anxiety. *Attacking Anxiety: A Proven Way to Regain Self-Control and Self-Confidence,* audiocassette program. Midwest Center, Oak Harbor, OH, 1995.

Miller, Emmett E. *Feeling Good: How to Stay Healthy.* Upper Saddle River, NJ: Spectrum Book, Prentice-Hall, 1978.

Pelletier, Kenneth R. *Mind as Healer; Mind as Slayer: A Holistic Approach to Preventing Stress Disorders.* New York: Delta, 1977.

Peurifoy, Reneau Z. *Anxiety, Phobias and Panic: Taking Charge and Conquering Fear—A Step-by-Step Program for Regaining Control of Your Life.* East Longmeadow, MA: Lifeskills, 1988.

Seligman, Martin E. *What You Can Change and What You Can't: The Complete Guide to Successful Self-Improvement.* New York: Fawcett Columbine, Ballantine Books, 1993.

Vaillant, George. *Adaptation to Life.* Boston: Little, Brown, 1977.

Vayda, William. *Mood Foods: How the Foods We Eat Affect Our Emotions, Moods, and Personality.* Berkeley, CA: Ulysses Press, 1995.

Ward, Berbard. *Think Yourself Well: The Amazing Power of Your Mind.* New York: Globe Communications, 1995.

Wilson, R. Reid. *Don't Panic: Taking Control of Anxiety Attacks.* New York: Harper & Row, 1986.

Wooten, Patty. *Compassionate Laughter: Jest for Your Health.* Salt Lake City, UT: Commune-A-Kay, 1996.

Wurtman, Judith J. *Managing Your Mind and Mood Through Food.* New York: Harper Perennial, 1988.

Beverly A. Potter, Ph.D., received her doctorate in counseling psychology from Stanford University and her master's degree in vocational rehabilitation counseling from San Francisco State University.

Docpotter is noted for challenging rules and thinking of issues from a fresh perspective. She blends philosophies of humanistic psychology, social learning theory, and Eastern philosophies to create an inspiring and original approach to handling the challenges we encounter today.

Docpotter is a recognized authority on how to overcome job burnout. She provides keynote speeches and training for associations and corporations. Her offices are in Oakland, California. Please visit her website at www.docpotter.com.

CPSIA information can be obtained at www.ICGtesting.com
Printed in the USA
BVOW11s2229270915

419821BV00010B/157/P